Nutrition and Exercise in Obesity Management

SPORTS MEDICINE AND HEALTH SCIENCE

Philip K. Wilson, Ed D.
Senior Series Editor
Executive Director
La Crosse Exercise Program
University of Wisconsin-La Crosse

Henry S. Miller, M.D.
Associate Series Editor
Professor of Medicine-Cardiology
Bowman Grey School of Medicine,
Wake Forest University

Nutrition and Exercise in Obesity Management

Edited by

Jean Storlie, M.S., R.D.
Research Associate
Institute for Aerobics Research
Dallas, Texas

Henry A. Jordan, M.D.
Director
Institute for Behavioral Education
King of Prussia
Pennsylvania

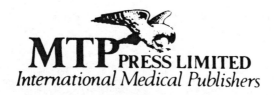
MTP PRESS LIMITED
International Medical Publishers

Published outside the western hemisphere by
MTP Press Limited
Falcon House
Lancaster, England

Published in the US by
SPECTRUM PUBLICATIONS, INC.
175-20 Wexford Terrace
Jamaica, NY 11432

ISBN 978-94-011-6721-5   ISBN 978-94-011-6719-2 (eBook)
DOI 10.1007/978-94-011-6719-2

Contributors

Elizabeth A. Ardito, M.S.   Obesity and Risk Factor Program, Wayne State University, Detroit, Michigan

Merle L. Foss, Ph.D.   Department of Physical Education, University of Michigan, Ann Arbor, Michigan

Barry A. Franklin, Ph.D.   Director, Cardiac Rehabilitation, Sinai Hospital of Detroit, Detroit, Michigan

Patricia Hodgson, M.S., R.D.   Cardiovascular Nutritionist, Mayo Clinic, Rochester, Minnesota

Nan Holmes, Ph.D.   Obesity and Risk Factor Program, Wayne State University, Detroit, Michigan

Charles P. Lucas, M.D.   Obesity and Risk Factor Program, Harper-Grace Hospitals; Department of Internal Medicine, School of Medicine, Wayne State University, Detroit, Michigan

Michele Macedonio, M.S., R.D.   Director, Nutrition Services, Thomas B. Guilliam Associates, Twinsburg, Ohio

Dallas Stevenson, M.S.   Clinical Psychologist, Obesity and Risk Factor Program, Wayne State University, Detroit, Michigan

Deborah A. Strehle   Fitness Director, Westside Tennis and Fitness Club, Little Rock, Arkansas

Contents

Foreword

It is a pleasure to present, *Nutrition and Exercise in Obesity Management*, for reference and textbook use. The text is an outgrowth of the Obesity-Weight Control Track of the 1982 La Crosse Health and Sports Science Symposium, sponsored annually by the La Crosse Exercise Program, University of Wisconsin-La Crosse. With versatile faculty, topics, and attending professionals, the Obesity-Weight Control Track stimulated an effort to produce interdisciplinary resources on obesity.

Out of this effort, three books have been compiled and edited. The first book, *Evaluation and Treatment of Obesity*, introduces an interdisciplinary, practical approach to obesity management. This book, *Nutrition and Exercise in Obesity Management*, compiles the information specifically related to nutrition and exercise management of obese individuals. The third book, *Behavioral Management of Obesity*, relates behavioral theories to the modification of eating habits and activity patterns. These three books apply the latest information from the fields of medicine, nutrition, exercise, and psychology to the problem of obesity. The information is intended to guide health professionals in the interdisciplinary management of obesity.

In 1983 the Obesity-Weight Control Track focused on controversial issues of theoretical and practical concern. The speakers from this track contributed their expertise to the compilation of two additional books. Thus, *Trends and Controversies in Obesity Research* and *Innovation in Obesity Program Development* will complete the series. Consider the five volumes a consolidated, comprehensive reference related to the growing, interdisciplinary field of weight control.

The co-editors and individual chapter authors of this book, and the entire series, should be complimented for providing the practicing health professional with a valuable book. Researching and writing this material has been enlightening and exciting to those involved; we trust its value to you will be similar.

Philip K. Wilson, Ed.D., Senior Series Editor
Henry Miller, M.D., Associate Series Editor

Introduction

Nutrition and Exercise in Obesity Management is one book of a five part series on obesity. The entire series is intended to (1) provide an understanding of the multiple factors that influence human obesity, and (2) apply this knowledge in developing comprehensive, rational approaches to weight management. A number of professional disciplines have made valuable contributions to the current understanding of human obesity. It is our belief that the complexities of this condition require the cooperation between and coordination of all these professions. Although the content of this series is divided into five books, it should be recognized that the material is interrelated and interdependent.

Consistent with this philosophy, the first volume in this series, *Evaluation and Treatment of Obesity*, approaches obesity management from an interdisciplinary perspective. Concepts related to dietary management and physical activity are expanded upon in *Nutrition and Exercise in Obesity Management*, while *Behavioral Management of Obesity* elaborates on the behavioral theories and practices. The last two books, *Trends and Controversies in Obesity Research*, and *Innovation in Obesity Program Development*, are intended to address current issues of theoretical and practical concern. Within this comprehensive framework, the entire series approaches basic concepts in light of the problems that face practitioners at the "cutting edge" of obesity research and intervention.

Nutrition and Exercise in Obesity Management presents practical techniques for solving the nutrition- and exercise-related problems of obese individuals. Chapter 1 critiques popular diet plans in relation to sound principles of nutrition. Chapter 2 provides guidelines and procedures for establishing nutrition care practices. Chapter 3 considers the protein-sparing modified fast as a therapeutic adjunct to interdisciplinary behavioral management. The three chapters on exercise, Chapters 4, 5, and 6, apply principles of fitness and exercise physiology to weight control programming. Practical concerns related to prevalent myths and important precautions are examined.

The authors contribute not only their theoretical knowledge, but also knowledge based on considerable experience working with obese individuals. An attempt has been made to present theories, describe the practical applications, and discuss the "gaps" between theory and practice. This approach is intended to stimulate growth and innovation on the part of health professionals using this resource.

We hope that this book, and the entire series, will encourage health care professionals to face the problem of obesity intervention with practical and theoretical tools, as well as an interdisciplinary attitude. This effort can provide safe and rational alternatives to the myriad of untested, unscientific, at times unsafe, and ineffective programs that abound in our society.

Jean Storlie, M.S., R.D.
Henry A. Jordan, M.D.

Contents

1

Review of Popular Diets

Patricia Hodgson

INTRODUCTION

Individuals in our society are obsessed about their weight.
For many, daily feelings (miserable or ecstatic) are determined
at the moment of the morning ritual of stepping on the scale.
As a consequence, Americans are searching for weight-reducing
methods. What they find are a few methods that are bona fide
and many that are worthless.

George Bernard Shaw noted that medical practice is governed
not by science but by supply and demand [1]. The grossest
quackery cannot be kept off the market if there is a demand for
it, and there is nothing more in demand than quick, easy, and
painless weight loss. Popular fad diets thus cater to the tastes
of the public.

The medical profession has long considered excess weight an
emotional, generally incurable disorder. Thus it has no official

standards for treating overweight individuals, partly because being fat is not itself an illness [2]. With the medical profession being inherently disinterested, physicians tend to treat this disorder in a casual manner giving out archaic advice. Consequently, the success rate for weight reduction is dismal. Even those physicians with expertise and interest in treating overweight have not devised a sure-proof method for weight control.

The bottom line, however, is frustrated, desperate dieters who turn to nonmedical methods to become thinner. These methods often fall into the realm of the bizarre. Generally useless and sometimes dangerous, the problem is that lay persons do not have the knowledge to discriminate between good and bad methods, between safe or hazardous regimens.

The government agency responsible for the safety of food and appropriate labeling, the Food and Drug Administration, is not permitted to regulate claims issued by proponents of dietary regimens unless a book or article is used to misbrand a particular food [3]. For example, when Dr. Herman Taller promoted safflower oil as a fat-burning substance in his book *Calories Don't Count* [4], the FDA had the right to step in because the book's sales were tied in with that of safflower oil capsules.

For the most part, claims made in articles and books for foods or weight-loss regimens are not under the jurisdiction of this government agency. Because the First Amendment to the Constitution safeguards freedom of speech, anyone, regardless of background, can publish extravagant claims in the lay press. Unless the safety of food or its labeling is involved, charlatans can promote nostrums and nonsense openly and without fear of prosecution.

Dr. Edward Rynearson, in an article entitled "Americans Love Hogwash," outlined various examples of food faddism and their proponents [5]. He encouraged the medical profession to protect patients from unscientific weight loss faddism by themselves being aware of dietary "hogwash" and being able to give knowledgeable advice to individuals requesting information.

Numerous diet schemes have been devised since civilization began. Probably one of the early ones was Pliny's advice in

114 AD that "Simple diet is best, for many dishes bring many diseases." Diet books are among the most popular literature on the market. The best sellers list of nonfiction books frequently has a diet book mentioned in the top ten.

Each year over 100 articles on diets will appear in lay magazines. The average American may go on and off 1½ diets per year [6]. Fifty-three percent of the adult population surveyed in 1980 reported efforts to control weight [7], and at any given time 20% of the population are on some kind of weight-loss program [8]. Each week over one million people participate in group weight-loss programs. The diet industry generates at least $10 billion yearly with over $75 million spent on appetite suppressant drugs alone [9]. Past and current diet mania reflect Americans' obsession over weight problems and our passion for being lean and slim.

If any of these diets worked, new ones would not have to be devised. Why do these diet schemes fail? People in this day and age have unrealistic expectations of weight losses because of advertisements for quick weight-loss gimmicks. The advertisements promise fast, quick, and painless results. People are willing to try anything that sounds simple. Immediate gratification of a desire is a characteristic of our society. People have been spoiled by affluence, purchasing what is desired without having to wait for any length of time. An overweight individual told by a registered dietitian that a 1- to 2-pound loss per week is realistic and thus it may take 6 months to 1 year to lose 50 pounds on a balanced low-calorie diet is not in the habit of waiting so long for a wish to be granted. Instead, a faster way to lose is sought.

Our society also is accustomed to a full stomach. Having to forego feelings of fullness after meals and pleasures of frequent snacks when desired is a sacrifice most have not had to endure. In our society with its abundance and varieties of food, eating what one desires is considered an inalienable right. Thus people seek the perfect diet, i.e., the one where weight loss is promised while eating and drinking as much as desired without having to exercise.

GUIDELINES FOR EVALUATING DIETS

Ways of evaluating diets have been devised. The *Consumer Guide* has been publishing a paperback called "Rating the Diets" [10]. In the current edition over 100 diets are evaluated. The following guidelines in evaluating weight-loss schemes are used:

1. Has the author of the diet tried the regimen on hundreds, even thousands, of overweight people and objectively compared the results against a similar number of controls on regular or other weight-reducing diets and published the findings in a recognized and reputable medical journal? If the answer is no, regard the diet experimental at best.

2. Is the person promoting the diet known, well-respected, and knowledgeable in nutrition? Many physicians have published books on diets, but simply being a physician does not qualify one in nutrition.

3. How long has the diet been around? If less than five years, view it with suspicion. Anyone can invent a new diet, but only a few diets survive. At the same time, many old diets which tend to be regularly resurrected should have been laid to eternal rest.

4. Is the proponent of the new diet challenging the recommendations of bona fide experts? If it is a valid challenge, it should be backed by substantial scientific data.

5. Does the diet regimen allow for individual preference, practice, and taste? Rigid diets that tell the dieter what and when to eat are doomed to fail in the long run because it does not allow flexibility to follow the rhythm of life activities.

6. Is the diet based on principles of another expert or health association? If so, what is the opinion of the individuals or organization about the regimen? Numerous diet regimens have been based on outside research. The original proponent often is not consulted and may not approve of the regimen if allowed to have input.

7. In looking at the diet itself, is the diet based on some "secret" no one has discovered before? Is it limited to a few foods? Does it stress expensive or unusual foods? Does it warn

against eating a combination of foods at one time? Does it omit foods of high nutritional value such as dairy products, breads, and other grains? Does it depend on vitamin and mineral concentrates to balance the diet? Does the author warn of any side effects or special precautions? Does the regimen include increased exercise?

8. Could the dieter live on the regimen for the rest of his or her life? Since weight control is a full-time, lifelong effort, individuals need to develop good eating habits as the weight is lost.

To apply these guidelines to the analysis of two diets, I now evaluate "Easy-Does-It" Wise Woman's Diet and the Beverly Hills Diet according to these eight criteria.

The "Easy-Does-It" Wise Woman's Diet meets most of the guidelines of *Consumer Guides* "How to Rate a Diet." It is a 1200-calorie diet originally devised by two physicians who are experts in nutrition, Dr. Norman Jellife and Dr. George Cristakis. It has been published in *Redbook Magazine* two to three times each year since 1967. A recent revised version was prepared by three recognized experts in nutrition and weight control: Dr. Johanna Dwyer from the New England Medical Center Hospital, Dr. Jules Hirsch from the Rockefeller University Hospital, and Dr. Myron Winick from Columbia University [11]. The diet is well-balanced, includes a variety of foods, and does not depend on any secret for its success. It is the type of regimen that one could easily live with for a lifetime, and no one is making a lot of money promoting it.

In contrast to this safe and durable way to lose weight is the Beverly Hills Diet promoted by Judy Mazel, a self-styled non-nutritionist [12]. After being on the nonfiction best seller's list for several weeks in 1981, its demise occurred several months later after she had made a fortune on the sale of her book. Basically it is a low-calorie fruit diet. For the first week the dieter eats only fruit: papaya, mango, strawberries, apricots, blueberries, watermelon, apples, and prunes. On the eleventh day bagles, butter, and corn on the cob are allowed, and not until the nineteenth day is protein permitted in the form of steak or lobster. Then through the fifth week, protein foods are permitted one day a week.

The Beverly Hills Diet is based on the secret discovered by the author that enzymes in fruit can render other foods less fattening and that protein and carbohydrate digestive enzymes cannot work together. In all respect, this diet does not meet any of the guidelines suggested by *Consumer Guide*.

Diets that fall in this same category are the Scarsdale Diet, the Last Chance Diet, the Quick Weight Loss Diet, plus hundreds of others including the Stillman Diet which started the diet mania vogue in 1960 [10]. This diet, also called the Drinking Man's Diet, is another one of the high-protein, low-carbohydrate regimens. The appeal of this and other diets including the Beverly Hills Diet is rapid weight loss in a short period of time [10]. Nutrition experts quickly note that the weight lost is primarily water which the body replenishes as soon as normal eating resumes.

MOTIVATION TO FOLLOW FAD DIETS

A perplexing question is why people follow such programs which are completely adverse to usual eating practices. In addition to motivation provided by rapid weight loss, such regimens are appealing to individuals because controlling intake of unfamiliar foods is easier than the willpower required to eat less of their usual food.

One of America's leading experts on obesity, Dr. Hilda Bruch, has made some interesting observations on dieting [13]. She stated that many overweight individuals prefer rather unusual diets that will bring observable results quickly. To them drastic, extraordinary diets are more acceptable than just a slight change in one's established habits; the great appeal of absurd fads and outlandish diets appears to be related to this. In her work with overweight individuals, she found monotonous, somewhat strange diets more effective than reasonable restrictions. She says it is the very strangeness that makes these diets effective. In essence, they take dieting out of the realm of ordinary living. A drastic change in diet can be psychologically desirable because eating unfamiliar foods is a visual reminder of weight loss efforts and indicates that dieting is serious business. In essence, strange diets say that the former eating habits were bad, and in order to lose weight, the habits and foods to achieve that goal must be dramatically different.

RECENT POPULAR FAD DIETS

Many popular fad diets meet the criteria of being dramatically different. In addition to the Beverly Hills Fruit Diet, other recent innovations are the Pritikin Longevity Program, the Cambridge Diet, the Scarsdale Diet, the Last Chance Diet, and the latest promotion, starch blockers.

Cambridge Diet

The Cambridge Diet, a revised version of the Metracal formula introduced in 1959, was devised by Dr. Alan Howard of Cambridge University, England [14]. It is an outgrowth of his work with extremely low-calorie formulas for weight loss. The powdered formula comes in a can which costs $19.00 and lasts about one week. For the first three weeks an individual consumes only formula, one cup per meal, which daily provides 330 calories and 33 g of high quality protein. It comes in a variety of flavors including Hearty Chicken Soup and Double Dutch Chocolate Drink. After three weeks, a maintenance diet is followed for one week consisting of one meal per day and two servings of formula. Instructions are given that the formula diet is intended to be temporary.

The problem with this and other formula diets is that it does not educate the individual in good and poor eating habits. Followers of the program will never learn what food habits caused the weight problem and how to change them. Also, sudden and radical changes in diet such as a formula can be dangerous for individuals with undiagnosed diabetes, GI troubles, liver or kidney diseases, anemia, or some heart conditions. Ketosis is a common occurrence with extremely low-calorie regimens [10]. The American Dietetic Association released a statement to the media on August 19 "that the 330 Calorie-A-Day diet is not a common sense approach to weight loss and should not be undertaken without strict monitoring by a medical professional."

Last Chance Diet

A prime example of dangerous formula diets was the Last Chance Diet which used a liquid protein formula as the only source of calories [15]. Seventeen deaths of dieters were attributed to the use of the liquid protein formula.

Pritikin Maximum Weight Loss Diet

The Pritikin Program was developed specifically to help patients with heart disease, diabetes, hypertension, and gout. In the book *The Pritikin Program For Diet And Exercise*, two diets are outlined by Nathan Pritikin, founder and director of the Longevity Center in California [16], the Longevity Diet and the Maximum Weight Loss Diet. The former is not designed to reduce weight. Because it is low in fat, cholesterol, protein, and highly refined carbohydrates, the Longevity Diet may produce weight loss.

The Maximum Weight Loss Diet, also low in the above nutrients, outlines two calorie levels—600 calories and 1000 calories. The diets contain approximately 80% complex carbohydrate calories, 10% protein, and 10% fat. The 600 calorie regimen is basically a vegetarian diet whereas the 1000 calorie diet allows one serving of fish or fowl every other day, not to exceed 1½ pounds per week. Dieters are encouraged to eat large quantities of vegetables and to "eat all day." Exercise, an important component of any weight reduction regimen, is an integral part of the Pritikin Program. The statement is made that "Exercise must have top priority, one that supersedes everything except your spouse, your children, and the food you eat" [16].

The scientific community is divided in its assessment of the Pritikin Plan [17]. Some see it as nutritionally sound and useful while others criticize it as restrictive and austere. The American Medical Association questions the safety and effectiveness of the program in respect to the diseases it is supposed to prevent [3].

The Scarsdale Diet

The Scarsdale Medical 14-Day Diet appeared in 1978 and is still popular [18]. Essentially this diet is another one of the high-protein, low-carbohydrate diets that continually reappear in revised versions. The diet contains 43 percent protein compared to 12 percent recommended by various health professionals, 22.5 percent fat, and 34.5 percent carbohydrate and totals 1000 calories per day. Dr. Herman Tarnower, the author, claimed one-pound loss per day and wisely recommended that the diet be adhered to no longer than 14 days. The reason for its success, according to Dr. Phillip White, secretary of the Council on Foods and Nutrition of the AMA, was its extreme rigidity [9]. The dieter had few decisions to make, encouraging compliance. Other attributes were that it stressed a high protein intake, a nutrient considered as a status symbol in this country. For example, two days a week the dieter is encouraged to eat "plenty of steak" without indicating quantity. Another positive trait was that the diet was named after a symbol of success, the community of Scarsdale, one of the richest in the U.S.

The diet's rigidity is reflected in its rules: Eat only foods listed on the carefully planned 14-day menu, make no substitutions, never overload the stomach, and do not stay on it for longer than 14 days. For two weeks the dieter follows the Keep Trim Eating Plan, allowing for a wider variety of foods. Dieters do not have to think because menus are preplanned. The Scarsdale Diet will cause weight loss temporarily, but like all such regimens dieters do not learn good eating habits necessary for weight maintenance.

Nutritionally, the diet is low in calcium; dairy products are allowed only on Friday. It also does not specify quantities of food but instead gives dieters unrestricted amounts such as "eat all you want of fruit salad" for Tuesday's lunch and "plenty of steak" for Tuesday's and Friday's dinner. Lack of restriction on amounts are given may be another reason why the program appeals to millions of people. However, one reason why people are overweight is because they eat too much in relation to what they expend and probably the last thing they need is the freedom to misuse or abuse food portions.

Starch Blockers

Because so many popular fad diets discourage carbohydrate consumption, the American public has misconceptions about this nutrient, considering it high calorie. When starch blockers were introduced in 1982, the dieting public was ecstatic. Over 200 manufacturers aggressively marketed starch blockers as the answer to the dieter's prayers. Because it contained an enzyme from kidney beans which purportedly prevented digestion and absorption of starch, advertisements announced that individuals could eat ad libitum of pasta, bread, pizza, etc., and not gain weight. However, numerous side effects were noted with the pill such as nausea, vomiting, abdominal cramps, and diarrhea. Hospitalization was required in several cases [19].

In the fall of 1982, the Food and Drug Administration banned the sale of starch blockers until further studies could be performed. Although numerous studies reportedly have been conducted showing weight loss as a result of taking starch blockers, these studies have not been published. This is another example of a gimmick and, like all gimmicks, it will go away. That is true of most fad diets; eventually they fade away.

POPULAR COMMERCIAL WEIGHT LOSS CLINICS

Commercial weight loss clinics, coming to the aid of dieters, are big business. People find in these clinics the magic ingredient missing in diets from a book, Tender Loving Care or TLC.

Various nutrition experts agree that diet groups are helpful for some people, particularly those who are mildly to moderately overweight [20,21]. The key element with each group is the external support from the leader and other members and the exposure to successful models. Evangelistic spirit, peer pressure, group solidarity, and healthy competition are additional key elements. The self-help approach provided an effective mechanism for weight loss of obese persons. One of the keys to their success is that members regard each other as intelligent persons who have the power to overcome their eating problems if they so desire.

Weight Watchers

A well-known self-help group is Weight Watchers, an up-to-date, professionally backed commercial diet club that offers the latest techniques in weight control [10]. At some time during its 16-year history, more than 12 million people have made contact with the organization. Over 12,000 classes are held each week in the U.S. and 30 foreign countries.

Losing weight with Weight Watchers is not cheap. The dieter must pay a registration fee of around $10.00 and weekly meeting fees of $5.00. When a meeting is skipped, the fee for it has to be paid before additional ones can be attended. Weight Watchers feels that dieters should pay because the fees represent a commitment that will not be forgotten in a week or two. Weight Watchers' staff includes Dr. Reva Frankle, a well-known nutritionist; Dr. W. Henry Sebrell, a physician who was chief of nutrition at Columbia University; Dr. Lenore Zohman, a physician well-known in the area of exercise; and Dr. Richard Stuart, whose area of expertise is behavior modification techniques.

Weight Watchers' weight-loss program includes three aspects: diet, exercise, and behavior modification. In a study of 7,623 members, Stuart found an average weight loss of 1.6 pounds per week, 15 percent greater average weekly weight loss than for members who were on diet alone. Fifteen months later a study of 721 members of the experimental group showed that 50 percent were within 5 percent or less of their goal. To date, this study has not been published in a medical journal, but only reported at a meeting.

TOPS

If Weight Watchers does not do the trick, the dieter has numerous alternatives available. One is TOPS, or Take Off Pounds Sensibly, which was started in 1948. Initially, its key element was moral support from leaders and other group members. It does not provide an official diet, maintaining that members should receive a dietary program from a medical professional. TOPS does provide dietary guidelines based on the recommendations of the U.S. Senate Committee on Nutrition and Human Needs. In the book sold only to members, *A Nutrition Monograph For Taking Off Pounds Sensibly*, guidelines are indicated for three calorie levels—1200 calories, 1500 calories, 1800 calories [22].

There are five facets of TOPS—medical research into various aspects of obesity, medical supervision of members' diets, group therapy process with each chapter electing its leaders and conducting their own meetings, keen competition with special recognition given yearly to those who lose the most weight and instructions in behavior modification. Dr. Albert Stunkard compared weight losses of TOPS members with those reported in the medical literature [20]. He found that results were similar and concluded that these comparisons offer strong evidence of the effectiveness of TOPS.

Some organizations such as the Diet Center and Nutri-System differ from Weight Watchers and TOPS in that individuals are counseled on a one-to-one basis rather than in group sessions.

The Diet Center

The Diet Center advertisement says it is a "sensible weight loss program that really works" [10]. It works because it is rigid in type and amount of food; only about 17 foods are allowed. Probably its most important attribute is that the dieter is encouraged to weigh every day at the Center. The 750 calories per day is designed to cause 17–25 pounds weight loss during a six-week period. A diet supplement of B-vitamins is taken every four hours each day to alleviate stress caused by dieting. Probably the main benefit of taking pills frequently during the day is that it reminds the dieter every four hours of the weight loss goals. In addition, the dieter is encouraged to take supplementary calcium and vitamin C.

Proponents of the Diet Center indicate the diet is adequate in all essential nutrients; however, as nutrition experts know, it is difficult to plan a well-balanced diet on less than 1000 calories. The program encourages exercise, offers classes on behavior modification, and has a follow-up program of weekly weigh-ins for one year at no charge to encourage weight maintenance.

Nutri-System

Nutri-System also features individual sessions with dieters and weekly weigh-ins. In contrast to Diet Center, Nutri-System requires a medical exam by a physician and dieters have to buy almost all food consumed from the organization. These items are prepared and pre-portioned so clients do not have to make any choices. Jazzy names are given to the food such as Nebula Nectar (orange juice), Space Cakes (pancakes), Eggs Appolo, Lunar Crepes, and Nutri Flakes. Cost is $90.00 for the exam, $35.00 per week for the food, and $25.00 per week for the consultation and weigh-ins.

Criticism by the medical profession of esoteric diet regimens is applicable to Nutri-System. There is the possibility of ketosis, dehydration, significant intracellular losses of essential electro-lytes and nutrients, and the occurrence of rapid weight gain once the regimen is discontinued [10].

Evaluation of Commercial Weight Loss Clinics

An editorial in the April 1982 issue of *Archives of Internal Medicine,* by Dr. Tony Gotto from Baylor College of Medicine in Texas and an expert in weight control, stresses the importance of evaluating commercial clinics by outcome [24]. He suggests that, at a minimum, a clinic should provide data regarding drop out rate over time, average post-treatment weight loss and average weight loss at least one year after treatment ends.

Several points to consider when evaluating a clinic is whether treatment is preceded by careful medical and behavioral assessment, as well as collection of data on baseline eating patterns and prior attempts of weight loss. Because greater long-term success in weight reduction is found if a program includes an exercise component, physical activity should also be assessed. Unfortunately, most commercial clinics emphasize only decreased intake with little attention to increased activity.

During treatment, close medical supervision is essential and commitment to the program should last long enough for the patient's changes in eating and exercise behavior to become a natural part of lifestyle. Studies have found large attrition rates in some commercial clinics with 70–80 percent dropping out before an appreciable amount is lost [25]. Doctor Gotto suggests that a treatment program should counsel patients to overcome feelings of failure in case they do drop out. An individual needs to realize that dropping out of a program does not mean that he is a failure as a person, but that his lack of motivation to follow that particular regimen was the real cause of dropping out.

SUMMARY

Fad diets promising rapid, effortless weight loss will be popular as long as our society stresses a slender body, provides an overabundance of high-calorie foods, and discourages physical activity. Faith will forever reside not only in the heart, but also in the stomach, of the overweight that a magic formula will be discovered allowing eating and drinking abundantly at the same time that excess weight is being shed. However, Americans ultimately have to learn that patience is important for weight loss.

REFERENCES

1. Shaw, G. B. *The Doctor's Dilemma*. Penguin Books, Inc., Baltimore MD, 1974.
2. Bennett, W., and Gurin, J. *The Dieter's Dilemma*. Basic Books, Inc., New York, 1982.
3. Willis, J. *Diet Books Sell Well But* . . . . FDA Consumer, March 1982.
4. Taller, H. *Calories Don't Count*. Simon and Schuster, New York, 1961.
5. Rynearson, E. Americans love hogwash. *Nutrition Reviews*, Supplement, July, 1974.
6. Bayrd, E. *The Thin Game*. Avon, New York, 1978.
7. Benchmark National Survey, *Exercise-Nutrition-Health Habits*. Trost Associates Inc., April, 1981.
8. *Health United States, 1979*. U.S. Department of Health, Education and Welfare, Public Health Services, Office of Health Research, Statistics and Technology, DHEW Publications No. 80-1232, Washington, D.C.
9. Greenberg, I., Palambo, J., and Blackburn, G. Obesity: facts, fads, and fantasies. *Comprehensive Therapy* 5:68, 1979.
10. Berland, T. Diets '81—rating the diets. *Consumer Guide*, May, 1981.
11. Droyer, J. Easy-does-it wise woman's diet. *Redbook*, January, 1980.
12. Mazel, J. *The Beverly Hills Diet*. Macmillan Publishing Co. Inc., New York, 1981.
13. Bruch, H. *Eating Disorders*. Basic Books, Inc., New York, 1973.
14. Howard, A., Grant, A., Edwards, O., Littlewood, E., and Baird, I. M. The treatment of obesity with very-low-calorie liquid formula diet. *Int. J. Obesity* 2:321, 1978.
15. Linn, R., and Stuart, S. *The Last Chance Diet*. Lyle Stuart, Inc., Secaucus, N.J., 1976.
16. Pritikin, N., and McGrady, P. *The Pritikin Program For Diet And Exercise*. Grosset and Dunlap. Inc., New York, 1979.
17. Barnard, R., Weber, R., Weingarton, W., Bennett, C., and Pritikin, N. Effects of an intensive, short-term exercise and nutrition program on patients with coronary heart disease. *J. Card. Rehab.* 1:99, 1981.
18. Tarnower, H., and Baker, S. *The Complete Scarsdale Medical Diet*. Wade Publishers, Inc., 1978.
19. Block those starch blockers. *Time Magazine*, July 26, 1982.
20. Stunkard, A., Levine, H., and Fox, S. Study of a Patient Self-Help Group for Obesity. 122nd Annual Meeting of American Psychiatric Association, Miami, Florida, May, 1969.

21. Stuart, M., and Mitchell, C. Self-help groups in the control of body weight. In *Obesity*, A. Stunkard (ed.). W. B. Saunders, Philadelphia, 1980.
22. Kalkhoff, R. *A Nutrition Monograph For Taking Off Pounds Sensibly.* Milwaukee: TOPS Club, Inc., 1980.
23. Stunkard, A. The success of TOPS, a self-help group. *Post Graduate Medicine* May 1972, 143-147.
24. Gotto, A., and Goodrick, G. Evaluating commercial weight loss clinics. *Arch. Intern. Med. 42*:682, 1982.
25. Volkmar, F., Stunkard, A., Woolston, J., and Bailey, R. High attrition rates in commercial weight reduction programs. *Arch. Intern. Med. 141*:427, 1981.

2

Nutritional Management of the Obese Individual

Michele Macedonio

INTRODUCTION

Given the known and theorized physiological, psychological, and social/environmental factors affecting obesity, the clinician will best support the obese client when treatment is designed to modify as many factors as possible.* The purpose of this chapter is to provide a blueprint from which the clinician can design an individualized nutritional plan for weight control. Since permanent weight control requires a lifetime commitment to

---

*See M. Macedonio, Regulation of energy balance. In *Evaluation and Treatment of Obesity*, edited by J. Storlie and H. A. Jordan (New York: Spectrum Publications, 1984).

healthful eating and exercise behaviors, an efficacious plan is one which addresses the physiological, psychological, and social/environmental influences affecting the client.

A practical approach to developing a nutritional regimen is one which utilizes some basic management techniques. Throughout counseling, the dietitian should design and revise the program within the following cycle: (1) assessment, (2) problem identification and ranking, (3) designing and setting expected results (goals and objectives), (4) improvement strategy: the management plan, and (5) measurement/evaluation.

ASSESSMENT

In order to make an appropriate plan, it is crucial to perform a nutritional assessment. The assessment should provide as much information as the dietitian needs to help formulate realistic long and short term goals. Much of this information can be gathered via a client profile questionnaire (Figure 1) and a three day food intake record (Figure 2) completed by the client. Alone, an analysis of foods eaten over three days will not provide sufficient information upon which to base a comprehensive management plan. A client profile should fill in the gaps and expand upon this base. Questions detailing (1) the number of meals eaten, where they are eaten, how they are prepared; (2) the frequency of consumption of various foods, groups of foods, and food supplements; (3) beliefs about foods; (4) family and personal history of overweight; (5) occupation and workhours— all aid in drawing a more complete picture of a client's present eating behaviors. By asking questions about exercise habits and preferences, the dietitian further broadens the information base upon which a management plan is designed. Educational strategies and emphases can be tailored to the needs of the individual as evidenced in the assessment.

When available, a computerized analysis of food consumption can serve both as the basis for designing a dietary plan and as a tool for education. By combining anthropometric measurements and computer analysis of food intake, an objective data

Figure 1
PHYSICAL FITNESS TESTING CENTER
Patient Profile

Please answer all questions and record the amount of time it takes to complete this questionnaire.

1. Name _____

2. Present age _____ 3. Height _____ 4. Weight _____

   5. At age 20 _____ At age 30 _____ At age 40 _____

   One year ago _____ Most weighed _____

   Least weighed after age 20 _____ Desired weight _____

6. Pregnant? _____ Month _____ 7. Breastfeeding? _____

8. Vitamin/Mineral supplements _____
   (List and give reason for taking)

   _____

   On whose advice do you take vitamins? _____

9. Highest level of education <u>1 2 3 4 5 6 7 8 9 10 11 12 College</u> _____
   (Circle One)   (Years)

10. Employed ☐   Unemployed ☐   Retired ☐   Volunteer ☐

    Occupation _____

11. Business phone _____

12. Work hours _____ Full Time _____ Part Time _____

13. Single ☐   Married ☐   Widowed ☐   Separated ☐   Divorced ☐

14. Spouse: Employed ☐   Unemployed ☐   Retired ☐

    Occupation _____

Family History

15. Which members of your family are overweight?

    Father ☐   Mother ☐   Sisters ☐   Brothers ☐   None ☐

16. Favorite foods _____

17. Foods you do not eat _____

(continued)

Figure 1 *(Continued)*

18. Food allergies _____

19. Do you budget money for food? Yes ☐ No ☐ If so, approximate amount spent on food per week? _____

20. Number of persons living at home address _____

21. How many meals eaten/day? _____

22. Who does the cooking? _____

23. Which meals do you eat regularly?

    Breakfast _____   At what time? _____

    Lunch _____   At what time? _____

    Dinner _____   At what time? _____

24. What is your favorite meal? Breakfast ☐ Lunch ☐ Dinner ☐

25. What kinds of snacks do you eat? _____

    When? _____

26. What meals are eaten out?

    Breakfast   Times per week _____   Where? _____

    Lunch   Times per week _____   Where? _____

    Dinner   Times per week _____   Where? _____

    A. Restaurant B. Fast Food Restaurant C. Cafeteria D. Vending Machine
    E. Carry from home F. Home of friend/relative G. Other

27. What are the most important things to you at meal time?

    ☐ Eating the foods you like   ☐ Having enough food
    ☐ The way food is served   ☐ Someone to eat with and talk to
    ☐ The way food is cooked   ☐ Someone to cook
    ☐ Surroundings   ☐ Other (specify) _____

28. Is your appetite: Excellent ☐ Good ☐ Fair ☐ Poor ☐

29. Who does the shopping? _____

30. Is a shopping list used?   Yes ☐   No ☐

31. Are your meals planned? Yes ☐ No ☐ Weekly ☐ Daily ☐

Figure 1 *(Continued)*

32. Cooking facilities working: Refrigerator ☐ Range ☐ Oven ☐
    Broiler ☐ Freezer ☐ Microwave ☐

33. Indicate how often you use the following cooking methods.
    1 = Usually   2 = Occasionally   3 = Rarely   4 = Never

	Meats	Vegetables
Broiled	_____	_____
Fried	_____	_____
Baked	_____	_____
Boiled/Steamed	_____	_____
Roasted	_____	_____
Stewed	_____	_____
Microwaved	_____	_____
Uncooked	_____	_____

34. Do you regularly cook with fat? (oil, butter, margarine, lard, etc.)
    Yes ☐   No ☐

35. How many glasses of milk would you like to drink per day? 0 1 2 3 4
                                                           (Circle One)

36. Will you drink   Skim Milk   Yes ☐   No ☐
                           2%   Yes ☐   No ☐
                           1%   Yes ☐   No ☐
                    Whole Milk   Yes ☐   No ☐

37. Do you add salt to your food?   Yes ☐   No ☐
    If so, before tasting?   Yes ☐   No ☐   Heavy ☐   Medium ☐   Light ☐

38. Alcohol intake:
    Kind _____   Amount _____   Per _____
         _____   _____   _____
         _____   _____   _____

39. Which foods do you think are good for your health? _____
    _____

40. Which foods do you think are bad for your health? _____
    _____

41. Do you like to try new foods?   Yes ☐   No ☐

(continued)

Figure 1 *(continued)*

42. Do you use any "health" or "organic" foods?   Yes ☐ No ☐
     If so, what? _____

43. Are you on a special diet? Yes ☐ No ☐ If yes, what kind?_____

     _____

44. Do you have a chewing problem? Yes ☐ No ☐

45. Bowel Movements: Regular ☐ Irregular ☐

46. Do you take laxatives? Yes ☐ No ☐

47. If you take laxatives, how often? _____

48. How often do you eat these foods?

     Frequency of food use   Record as   Times/Wk   N - Never
                                               Times/Day   R - Rare

CHOLESTEROL: UNSATURATED FAT:
   Eggs   _____   Soft margarine   _____
   Liver   _____   Vegetable Oils   _____
   Shellfish   _____   SODIUM:
   Beef   _____   Prepared frozen foods _____
   Pork   _____   Sausages or franks   _____
   Cheese   _____   Snack foods, e.g.,
SATURATED FAT: pretzels, potato chips,
   Beef   _____   salted peanuts   _____
   Pork   _____   Softened Water   _____
   Butter   _____   Olives, pickles   _____
   Whole Milk   _____   Smoked fish,
   Cream   _____   canned fish   _____
   Pastries   _____   Ham & other
   Gravies   _____   canned meat   _____
   Ice Cream   _____   IRON:
SUGAR   Iron Supplements   _____
   Cakes   _____   Dark green leafy
   Pastries   _____   vegetables   _____
   Cookies   _____   Enriched cereals   _____
   Coke   _____   Dried Beans   _____
   Soda Pop   _____   Meat, fish, or
   Candy   _____   poultry   _____
                                      Eggs   _____

49. Did you have difficulty with any of the questions? No ☐ Yes ☐
     If yes, which one? _____
                        (Specify by numbers)

50. How long did it take you to complete this questionnaire? _____

Prepared by M. Macedonio, for Children's Hospital Medical Center of Akron, Ohio.

Figure 2
Three-Day Food Intake Record

PLEASE READ THESE INSTRUCTIONS CAREFULLY!

ACCURACY 1. This record will be computer analyzed. The accuracy of the nutritional analysis will depend on the degree of detail you provide in your food intake record. List everything you eat or drink for *three consecutive days,* under the column marked FOOD ITEM.
DO NOT CHANGE YOUR NORMAL EATING PATTERN OR HABITS DURING THIS TIME.

2. Under the column marked MEAL/SNACK, list whether that food was a part of a meal (B=Breakfast, L=Lunch, D=Dinner) or a between-meal snack (S=Snack).

AMOUNTS 3. Under the column marked AMOUNT, *precisely* record in household measures (level teaspoons, tablespoons, cups, or fractions of these) or in units such as one slice of bread, two eggs. When possible, *use measuring spoons and cups*, not tableware. In order for us to perform an accurate nutritional analysis, you must report exactly what you normally eat and drink.

ADDITIONS 4. Under the column, TYPE, COOKING METHOD, COMMENTS, record brand names, cooking method, and any other information about the food that may change its caloric or nutritional content; such as added condiments, butter, margarine, oil, gravies, sauces, toppings, dressings, breading, cream and sugar.

5. Consider the following: DETAIL IS CRITICAL!

Beverages
   A. State if whole, skim, 1%, 2%, buttermilk, powdered, evaporated, chocolate.
   B. FRUIT JUICES: List if fresh, frozen, canned or dehydrated; Record whether sweetened or unsweetened juice or drink.
   C. TEA, COFFEE: List amounts of sugar, cream, lemon, etc. under FOOD ITEM.
   D. DEHYDRATED: List brand name and liquid used if other than water.
   E. ALCOHOL: List the kind and amount of alcohol, (liquor, wine, beer, aperitif, cordial) and the kind and amount of mixer and other ingredients, (sugar, lemon, tonic, etc.)
   F. CARBONATED BEVERAGES: Specify with or without sugar and brand name.

(continued)

Figure 2 *(Continued)*

Breads
    A. Specify white, rye, whole wheat, raisin, biscuit, English muffin, bagel, etc. State if toasted.
    B. If butter, mayonnaise, jelly, etc. are added, list the kind and exact amount.
    C. Sandwiches: List ALL ingredients with the amounts (Bologna, lettuce, tomato, and mayonnaise).

Cereal
    A. Record the kind and amount in measuring cups or fractions of cups.
    B. If milk, sugar, fruits, etc. are added, list kind and amount.

Meat-Fish-Poultry — a small food scale will be helpful.
    A. List ounces or describe size (length, width, thickness; see illustration last page) in inches — after cooking, and without bone.

AFTER COOKING: 1 oz. = 2 TBSP. or a very small serving
                         3 oz. = 6 TBSP. or a small serving
                         4 oz. = 8 TBSP. or a medium serving

    B. Specify the cut of meat (ground chuck, top round steak, pork loin chop) and cooking method (baked, broiled, fried, etc.).
    C. List any breadings or batter.

Eggs
    A. Record cooking method as soft or hard cooked (boiled), poached, fried, scrambled, or omelet.
    B. If butter, milk, or drippings are used, specify the kind and amount.

Fruits and Vegetables
    A. Specify fresh, frozen, canned, dried, or freeze dried.
    B. Record COOKING METHOD as raw, fried, baked, simmered ("boiled"), etc.
    C. Fruits: list if canned in water, light syrup, heavy syrup, packed in its own juice, etc. If you drink the juice or syrup, record the amount.
    D. If butter, milk, cheese or bread crumbs are added, put kind and amount.

Desserts
    A. List commercial brand or "homemade" or "bakery".
    B. Bought candies and cookies: specify kind, size and brand name.

Figure 2 *(Continued)*

Desserts (continued)
- C. Pies: List size of pie pan (8" or 9") and what portion of pie you ate (1/8, 1/6, etc.).
- D. Cakes: List size (3" x 3", etc.). Specify one layer or two, type of icing or other topping. Brownies: Specify size, with or without icing, with or without nuts.
- E. Ice cream or frozen desserts: Specify whether ice cream or ice milk, sherbet, yogurt, soft ice cream, or frozen custard; list any toppings (nuts, sauces, cream)
- F. Cheesecake: Specify whether it has a fruit topping (fresh or canned).

Casseroles
- A. List if homemade, canned, or mix.
- B. Specify brand.
- C. Measure in cups.

Snack Foods
- A. Specify exact amounts, brand names, and food description. (Fritos Corn Chips, Doritos Tortilla Nacho Cheese Chips, Triscuits, Planter's Mixed Nuts Roasted with Oil).
- B. Popcorn: Specify if cooked with oil and whether butter is added.

MEAT SERVING SIZE GUIDE
(To Assist In Estimating Size of Meat Portions)

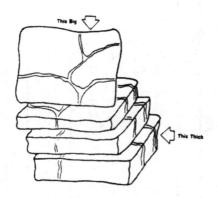

CHOOSE LEAN MEAT.
TRIM VISIBLE FAT.
BAKE, BROIL, ROAST,
STEW OR GRILL.
DISCARD FAT THAT
COOKS OUT OF MEAT.

MEAT: CALORIES PER OUNCE

1 oz. (or 30 grams) =	7 grams Protein +	3 grams Fat =	55 Calories
2 oz. (or 60 grams) =	14 grams Protein +	6 grams Fat =	110 Calories
3 oz. (or 90 grams) =	21 grams Protein +	9 grams Fat =	165 Calories

(continued)

Figure 2 *(Continued)*

DAY 1

NAME

MEAL/SNACK	FOOD ITEM	AMOUNT	TYPE, COOKING METHOD, COMMENTS
SAMPLE			
B	Rice Krispies	¾ cup	
B	Sugar	2 tsp.	
B	2% Milk	4 oz.	
B	Eggs	2	Fried in 1 Tbsp. bacon fat

NAME

DAY 2

MEAL/SNACK	FOOD ITEM	AMOUNT	TYPE, COOKING METHOD, COMMENTS

Prepared by M. Macedonio, for Children's Hospital Medical Center of Akron, Ohio.

Figure 3
Nutritional Assessment Summary

NAME _____ DATE _____

NUTRITIONAL ASSESSMENT IS BASED ON:

NUTRITIONAL ASSESSMENT
DATA BASE: Present Weight _____ Kg/ _____ Lbs
                Height _____ Cm/ _____ Ft _____ In.

                Computer Analysis of Patient Reported Three-Day
                Food Intake Record indicates daily averages of:

                Caloric Intake
                    Kilocalories (Kcal) _____ Kcal needed to maintain
                    present weight _____ /day

                Distribution of Kcal:
                    Protein _____ % Carbohydrate _____ %
                    Fat _____ % Alcohol _____ %/ _____ Kcal

                Recommended Distribution:
                    Protein _____ % Carbohydrate _____ %
                    Fat _____ %

                Cholesterol _____ mg Recommended (US Dietary
                Goals): < 300 mg/day

                Sodium _____ mEq + _____ tsp. salt= _____ mEq
                Recommended (RDA): < 150 mEq/day

                Nutrients consumed at levels less than two standard
                deviations of the mean (< 66-2/3%) of the RDA:

ANALYSIS:

Figure 3 *(Continued)*

ANALYSIS (Continued)

NUTRITIONAL PLAN

Desired Weight _____ Kg/ _____ Lbs

Recommended Weight _____ Kg/ ___ _____ Lbs

Goal: Weight _____ of _____ Kg/ _____ Lbs at the rate

of _____ Kg/ _____ Lbs per _____

_____

REGISTERED DIETITIAN

Prepared by M. Macedonio, for Children's Hospital Medical Center of Akron, Ohio.

base is formulated (Figure 3). Comparing kilocalories reported with those calculated to maintain present weight will aid the dietitian in setting a caloric deficit sufficient to support weight loss, yet close enough to the usual consumption so that adherence will be more likely. In anticipation of the plateauing phenomenon, kilocalories should be kept as high as possible while supporting weight loss. As a plateau is reached, kilocalories can be lowered to reinstitute a caloric deficit.

PROBLEM IDENTIFICATION AND RANKING

Based on the research implicating fat and simple carbohydrates as components of the diet which promote obesity, assessing the caloric distribution will indicate to the dietitian general problem areas. Comparing this information with actual foods consumed and usual frequencies, the prescribed diet can zero in on specifics. For example, if the client tends to eat significant amounts of meats, particular processed, cured and high fat meats, it can be pointed out that these are foods which raise the proportion of fat and cholesterol and should be limited. Carbohydrate can be divided into simple and complex carbohydrates. The dietitian, after identifying foods which provide generous amounts of either simple or complex carbohydrates, can make recommendations about increasing or decreasing particular foods based on their carbohydrate contribution. Scalfani and Springer's [1] work with supermarket diets provides strong support for minimizing high fat, high simple carbohydrate foods on a weight control program.* Sharing the results of these experiments with patients may provide cognitive motivation for altering food consumption patterns. Alcohol consumption is put into perspective when viewed as a percentage of kilocalories as well as absolute kilocalories per day. Once again, pointing out the caloric density and the nutrient paucity of alcohol may motivate the client to restrict or eliminate alcohol

---

*See M. Macedonio, Regulation of energy balance. In *Evaluation and Treatment of Obesity*, edited by J. Storlie and H. A. Jordan (New York, Spectrum Publications, 1984).

from the diet. Sodium content of the diet, when associated with particular foods rather than being narrowly limited to salt usage, provides the client with information necessary to modify another variable.

Overall, fats, sodium, and simple carbohydrates tend to concentrate in many of the same foods. Foods high in fat and simple carbohydrates do not usually contribute levels of vitamins and minerals commensurate with the amount of kilocalories; they are generally considered calorically dense and nutrient poor. A detailed nutritional assessment can be the initial vehicle for beginning a nutrition education program. By teaching the client which foods in his diet caused which nutrients to be consumed above or below recommended intakes, nutritional problems and recommendations for change become more objective, yet personalized. Once the problems are identified, they can then be ranked.

GOALS AND OBJECTIVES/MANAGEMENT PLAN/ MEASUREMENT AND EVALUATION

Each problem should have specific objectives. For example: Problem—the percentage of kilocalories as fat is higher than recommended. Dietary fats can be divided into visible (as in butter, margarine, oil, mayonnaise, salad dressing, cream, etc.) and hidden fats (as found in whole milk, fried foods, gravies, sauces, pastries, chips, and ice cream). An objective for change might be to assess a meal for visible and hidden fats. The strategy to meet the objectives could be keeping a food diary and the measurement is simple enough—was the diary kept? Once identifying fat in the diet becomes routine, a more advanced objective may be to limit the total amount of fat at each meal. A management plan for this objective could be menu planning. By setting forth the menu in advance, the client is more likely to stay within boundaries. Measurement once again can be made via the daily food diary.

To be successful, a weight management program must be tailored to the problem areas and needs of the individual client

and should have a strong educational component. Compliance
will be greater when the client understands the why and where-
fores of each step. Relating dietary modifications to physiologic
data such as serum cholesterol, triglycerides, blood pressure,
blood glucose, and percent body fat not only individualizes the
management plan, but provides a motivational impetus to alter
behavior and an objective measure of change. Time is well-spent
interpreting for clients the practical implications of current
research on weight control. For instance, by explaining the
metabolic adaptations which occur with weight plateauing, a
client is more likely to accept a higher, more sensible caloric
level and may be further motivated to engage in daily aerobic
exercise.

Two common situations may occur in a weight control program which, if not corrected, will inhibit the weight loss process.
First, clients will be overzealous. They have made up their
minds to lose weight and are actually disappointed, fearful,
"doubting Thomases" when given a kilocalorie level above
1,200 kilocalories. They know from past experience they will
never lose weight on a calorie level above 1,200! Second, some
patients will not have considered, nor are they willing to initiate,
an exercise component. They have no time, no desire, no facility
for exercise. Once again, an interpretation of the research
supporting not only the benefits of an exercise program, but the
fact that exercise helps prevent a drop in kilocalorie needs may
provide an objective motivator to follow the plan as outlined.

Realistic, achievable goals are essential in designing a work-
able plan. Reviewing and revising weight control plans with the
client teaches evaluation and decision-making skills which are
necessary parts to any dietary program. The consultant should
remember that the client always has the option of adopting or
rejecting advice, and that compromise may be needed in some
instances. If both counselor and client make the ultimate goal
a change in lifestyle, the result of which may be weight reduction, the treatment plan takes on a different focus. The imme-
diacy that accompanies quick weight loss schemes is neither
appropriate nor desirable. Rather, a one step at a time approach
allows the client to work on one problem until ready to tackle

another. For instance, getting someone who never eats breakfast to drink 8 ounces of juice is a start. What is considered traditional breakfast may be inappropriate for one person and ideal for another.

MEAL PLANNING

The role of the dietitian is to facilitate permanent change. Clients should be equipped with appropriate tools and raw materials to learn how to manage their diet and eating behaviors. The most important raw material in any weight control program is a simple, easy to use standard of food selection. One such standard is the Exchange List for Meal Planning designed by the American Dietetic Association and the American Diabetes Association. The versatility of the exchange system is broadened as the client learns not only the food list, but the basis for the groupings. This system is an ideal foundation for nutrition education. Although it does not provide for simple/refined carbohydrates, the dietitian can make adjustments when necessary. The more comprehensive the client's understanding of the exchange system, the better equipped they are to make informed choices.

Kilocalories needed to produce a caloric deficit should be based on kilocalories averaged over a three day period and/or an estimation of kilocalories needed to maintain present weight. A food nomogram [2] or a simple multiplication factor (e.g., weight in kilograms x 33) can be used to estimate caloric intake. If kilocalories are reduced 500 per day and exercise is increased to consume approximately 300 kilocalories per day 5 days per week, the caloric deficit would be 5,000 kilocalories per week. Since 3,500 kilocalories equal 1 pound of fat, it is reasonable to expect approximately a 1-1½ pound weight loss per week. A faster rate of weight loss can be achieved by decreasing the kilocalories further and/or increasing caloric expenditure through exercise. One advantage of a moderate reduction in caloric consumption coupled with a moderate increase in caloric expenditure is the ability to maintain moderate changes for

longer periods of time than if alterations are more drastic.
Actual food intake is often greater on a balanced, reduced
kilocalorie regimen if there is a shift from a high percentage of
fat and simple carbohydrates to a high percentage of complex
carbohydrates. Due to the caloric density of fats and sugars, this
alteration allows for larger quantities of food with fewer kilocalories. A common complaint of clients on a caloric distribution
of 50% carbohydrate, 20% protein, and 30% fat is that there is
too much food and they cannot consume all the allowed
exchanges!

TOOLS OF THE TRADE

The next step is to teach the client how to use the tools,
materials, and techniques of dietary management. What good is
a radial arm saw and wood to someone who knows nothing
about carpentry? Since humans learn best by doing, the dietitian
should help clients work for themselves. Menu planning is an
excellent technique for learning how to follow a meal pattern.
Once completed, menu plans become the blueprint of the diet.
Work sheets (Figure 4) provide a structure for menu planning
and reinforce the exchange system. Alterations in the original
plan can be made as needs change, but the base remains a
guiding thread. Providing the client with product information
further aids in the adjustment process.

A daily food record is an excellent weight management tool.
Recording makes clients aware of their food selection and its
frequency. Review of the food record teaches clients the
mechanics of the exchange system—how foods are grouped and
in what quantities they are measured. Suitable as a food record
is a steno pad, a small pocket pad, or even an elaborate sheet
detailing the location in which the food was eaten as well as the
stimulus to eat.

Inclusion of family members, whenever possible, reinforces
the educational process of weight management. Enlisting their
support and encouraging them is vital, for they, too, make
adjustments and sacrifices. The larger the social support system

DATE: _____

MEAL PLAN	EXCHANGES	BREAKFAST	snack	LUNCH:	snack	DINNER:	snack	# EXCH. ALLOWED	# EXCH. USED	GROCERY NOTES:
MILK	CHO 12 / Pro. 8 / Fat Trace / Kcal 80									
VEG.	CHO 5 / Pro. 2 / Fat – / Kcal 40									
FRUIT	CHO 10 / Pro. – / Fat – / Kcal 40									
BREAD	CHO 15 / Pro. 2 / Fat – / Kcal 70									
MEAT	CHO – / Pro. 7 / Fat 3 / Kcal 55									
FAT	CHO – / Pro. – / Fat 5 / Kcal 45									

Figure 4

Sample work sheet for menu planning. Prepared by M. Macedonio, for Children's Hospital Medical Center of Akron, Ohio.

a client has, the more successful the weight management program. Family and friends can be utilized in a "buddy system" technique. Patients are more likely to participate in an exercise program if accompanied by a friend, and the same principle applies to eating. As one woman asked, "How do you eat unbuttered popcorn as a snack while your husband eats a banana split?" This is an area where the dietitian must recognize "environmental sabotage" and trouble-shoot. There are situations in which environmental sabotage will be too great to overcome and it must be recognized that faced with such negative environmental forces, the client is not likely to follow through on weight loss.

By including "significant others" at the outset of counseling, potential problems may be avoided. For instance, prior to menu planning, asking family members to make a list of favorite meals and then including some of those meals in menu plans promotes a cooperative attitude. Teaching clients how to adjust recipes and reduce kilocalories without sacrificing taste is sure to please the dieter and his family. Providing new and taste-pleasing recipes which are simple to prepare is yet another technique for creating family support.

Teaching clients how to manage eating away from home is an essential part of counseling. In our modern society, most people eat in restaurants at least occasionally and have meals in the homes of family and friends as well. Preparing for eating away from home helps place more control over food selection in the hands of the client. That may mean taking along particular foods and beverages, eating part of a meal at home beforehand, saving exchanges from another meal to be eaten later, or increasing exercise to offset the extra kilocalories consumed.

In order to achieve and maintain a lower weight, caloric control and exercise must become a way of life. The weight loss portion of the management plan must be properly balanced and sustained for sufficient duration to affect a significant fat loss. An investigation by Benoit [3] of the composition of weight loss on a reducing regimen reports substantial fat losses as a result of fasting and a ketogenic diet. Perhaps due to misinterpretation of the data, a large part of the fat loss reported by

Table 1.   Nutritional Management Planning Scheme

I.   **Assessment**
   A.   Food intake analysis and nutritional assessment
   B.   Height/weight body composition

II.   **Problem identification**
   A.   Identify and rank problem areas of the diet, as evidenced in the nutritional assessment
   B.   Nutrition basics I
      1. Introduce the exchange system
      2. Define terms: calories, energy, carbohydrate, protein, fat

III. **Dietary structure**
   A.   Goal setting: long and short term goals and objectives
   B.   Meal pattern development

IV.   **Dietary revisions**
   A.   Evaluate goals and revise plan as necessary
   B.   Nutrition basics II: Integration of nutrition research and clinical management[a]
      1. Metabolic rate
         a) Effective caloric restriction
         b) Effective exercise
      2. Dietary factors
         a) One versus three or more meals per day
         b) Percentage of kilocalories as carbohydrate, protein, fat

V.   **Calorie costing**
         The exchange equivalent of recipes and convenience foods

VI.   **Menu planning**

VII. **Dining out**

VIII. **Incorporating fast foods into the exchange system**

IX.   **Brown-bagging it**

X.   **Entertaining for the health of it**

XI.   **Recipe adjustment and calorie reduction**

---

[a]See M. Macedonio, Regulation of energy balance. In *Evaluation and Treatment of Obesity*, edited by J. Storlie and H. A. Jordan (New York: Spectrum Publications, 1984).

38 MICHELE MACEDONIO

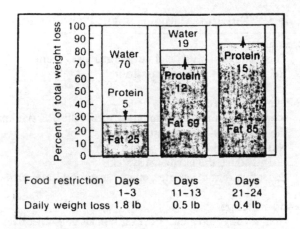

Figure 5. Percentage composition of weight loss at the start, middle, and end of 24 days of food restriction (1000 kcal per day) plus enforced exercise of 2.5 hours per day. From *Techniques for Measuring Body Composition*, National Academy of Sciences–National Research Council, Washington, D.C., 1961 (as cited in McArdle, W., Katch, F., and Katch, V., *Exercise Physiology*, Lea and Febiger, Philadelphia, 1981).

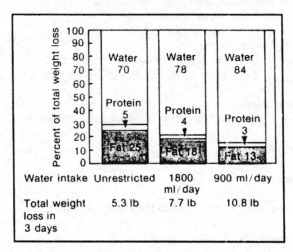

Figure 6. Percentage composition of weight loss during the first 3 days on a 1000-kcal carbohydrate diet with water intake unrestricted and reduced to 1800 ml and 900 ml per day. From *Techniques for Measuring Body Composition*, National Academy of Sciences–National Research Council, Washington, D.C., 1961 (as cited in McArdle, W., Katch, F., and Katch, V., *Exercise Physiology*, Lea and Febiger, Philadelphia, 1981).

Benoit and his colleagues was actually water loss. When insufficient dietary carbohydrate is available for fat metabolism, lean mass will be metabolized at a greater rate.

A study by Passmore, Strong, and Ritchie [4] analyzed the composition of obesity tissue during weight reduction. In a six-week period of weight loss, fat loss ranged between 73–83% of the loss, protein 4–7%, and water 10–23%. Initially, a labile portion of water was readily lost during the first few days on a reducing regimen. Figures 5 and 6 illustrate the shift in the composition of obesity tissue lost during weight reduction. Within the first three days, 70% of the loss can be attributed to water, 25% fat, and 5% protein. After three weeks of caloric restriction plus exercise, fat accounts for approximately 85% of the loss, 15% from protein. Continued weight reduction leads to a greater loss of fat per unit of weight loss. This data provides one more reason for clients to work toward a long term weight control program which combines controlled calories and increased exercise.

Table 1 is a suggested outline for planning nutritional management of a weight control program. It should be modified and expanded to meet the needs of each client.

At scheduled intervals, measurement and evaluation of goals and objectives should be made to assess behavior changes. The food diary can be effectively utilized throughout a weight control program as an evaluation tool.

CONCLUSIONS AND SUMMARY

Weight control is governed largely by physiological, psychological, social/environmental, dietary, and exercise factors. For a weight control program to be most effective [5,6], management should be comprehensive and thus, multidisiplinary involving physician, dietitian, mental health professional, and exercise physiologist. Education geared at a healthful lifestyle should be the basis for a weight management plan. The plan should be developed from long and short term goals which are realistic and achievable and based upon objective dietary, anthropmetric, and physiologic data. Review and revision are necessary to shape the management plan to the needs of the individual. Materials, tools and techniques are all critical components of a program designed to facilitate informed choice. The support and encouragement of the social environment should be nurtured and capitalized upon because of its pivotal role in this process of change. Not everyone can achieve "the body beautiful," but anyone can improve the quality of his life and raise his level of fitness through the adoption of a more healthful lifestyle. You don't have to be sick to get better! By these criteria, "successful" treatment of obesity is no longer an elusive ideal, but an achievable goal.

REFERENCES

1. Scalfani, A., and Springer, D. Dietary obesity in adult rats: similarities to hypothalmic and human obesity syndromes. *Physiol. Behavior 17*: 461–471, 1976.
2. Rynearson, E. H., and Gastineau, C. F. *Obesity*. Springfield, Ill.: Charles C Thomas, 1949.
3. Benoit, F. L., Martin, R. L., and Watten, R. H. Changes in body composition during weight reduction in obesity. *Ann. Inter. Medicine 61* (4):604–612, 1965.
4. Passmore, R., Strong, J. A., and Ritchie, F. J. The chemical composition of tissue lost by obese patients on a reducing regimen. *Br. J. Nutr. 12*:113–122, 1958.
5. American College of Sports Medicine. Position statement on proper and improper weight loss program. *Med Sci. in Sports and Exercise 15*:ix–xiii, 1983.
6. Tobias, A. L., and Gordon, J. B. Social consequences of obesity. *J. Amer. Diet. Assoc. 76*:338–342, 1980.

3

Protein-Sparing Modified Fasting and Behavior Therapy

Dallas Stevenson, Charles P. Lucas, Nan Holmes, and Elizabeth A. Ardito

INTRODUCTION

In reviewing the behavioral treatment of obesity Stunkard concluded that behavior therapy has advanced the treatment of this disorder, but might produce more clinically significant results if combined with other medical therapies [1]. One of the most promising new medical therapies is the protein-sparing modified fast (PSMF). Properly administered, this technique offers safe, rapid weight loss. What follows is a description of the various medical aspects of PSMF and its use in conjunction with behavior therapy as a treatment for obesity.

Genuth and Vertes introduced PSMF consisting of a small amount of carbohydrate added to a protein of high biological value [2]. While casein was used as the original protein source, more recently a commercial preparation has been employed, containing 300–400 calories, in which egg albumin is substituted for casein. Blackburn also developed a PSMF, consisting of 400–500 calories of lean beef, chicken, or fish per day [3]. It, like the PSMF of Genuth and Vertes, is supplemented with minerals and vitamins.

NITROGEN BALANCE

In order to ascertain the safety of PSMFs, several nitrogen balance studies have been conducted in subjects undertaking this regimen. Apfelbaum studied 41 females on a diet consisting only of 55 grams of protein. His patients lost an average of 21.9 grams of nitrogen in 19 continuous days of analysis [4]. Genuth found that individuals on a diet consisting of 70 grams of protein and 30 grams of carbohydrate (400 calories) had less than one gram of negative nitrogen balance daily after several weeks of diet [5]. Marliss followed nitrogen balance in six females and one male on a diet of only 83 grams of protein, and found nitrogen balance to be in equilibrium by the 12th day; and that cumulative nitrogen balance equalled –29 grams in 21 days of dietary therapy [6]. Bistrian et al. studied individuals who had been on a 300–400 calorie protein diet for several weeks, and found that these individuals could maintain nitrogen balance on 1.4 grams of protein per kilogram of body weight per day [7]. Fisler and Drennick studied the effects of various modifications of fasting on nitrogen balance in 40 subjects divided into four treatment groups [8]. Cumulative negative nitrogen balance averaged 186 grams for a group who were on a total fast, and 161 grams for the group on total fast given potassium chloride. The group given a low quality protein to supplement the fast had a cumulative negative nitrogen balance averaging 124 grams. When a high quality protein was used to supplement the fast, cumulative negative nitrogen balance averaged 102 grams. Other studies have not shown this high magnitude of negative nitrogen balance [6,7]. The larger negative balance observed by Fishler and Drennick may be attributed to the unique sample which consisted of males. In conclusion, there is evidence that PSMF can produce rather large losses of nitrogen over a prolonged period of modified fasting. Blackburn has suggested that this loss can be ameliorated by the use of 1.4 grams of protein per kg of body weight per day [7].

BLOOD CHEMISTRIES AND ELECTROLYTES

With rare exceptions, serum glucose, potassium, sodium, chloride, bicarbonate, and blood urea nitrogen remain normal for up to one year of PSMF. Serum uric acid frequently rises above 10 mg/dl over the first few weeks of PSMF, and later decreases into the 6–9 mg/dl range. Rare instances of gouty arthritis have resulted, which respond promptly to *colchicine* or *incomethacin*; and recurrent attacks are managed with chronic colchicine therapy. A transient increase in liver enzymes (SGOT, SGPT, alkaline phosphatase) has been observed in a notable percentage of patients within the first 2–4 weeks of PSMF. The increase is usually followed by a decline toward normal in most instances.

SIDE EFFECTS

Throughout PSMF there is a progressive decrease in blood pressure, even in normotensive subjects. This is associated with a decline in blood levels of catecholamines, and with negative sodium balance that occurs during the first week of PSMF. In some instances postural hypotension develops, but this rarely reaches clinical significance, and can be managed by adding salt (bouillon) and/or carbohydrate (sucrose) to the PSMF. Additional side effects include an early appearing skin rash, usually clearing after 1–2 weeks; fatigue and decreased mentation, which usually respond to an increase in the amount of protein; and hair loss, which can lead to considerable alopecia. Hair lost throughout the PSMF, returns to normal within 3–4 months of assuming an eucaloric diet.

Two other side effects of PSMF are worthy of comment. One is the rather frequent occurrence of cholecystitis observed during PSMF, often occurring 1–2 hours after patients violate the "fast" by eating food that contains fat. In view of the fact that gall stones and gall bladder colic are frequent in obese individuals, it is difficult to be certain that such attacks are provoked by PSMF. Such episodes are usually mild; however, in a number of instances they have led to elective cholycystectomy. The second side effect is the rare occurrence of foot drop, secondary to peroneal nerve neuropathy. The cause of this phenomenon is unknown. There is speculation that it is due to pressure on the peroneal nerve caused by patients crossing their legs. We have observed only one occurrence of foot drop in over 1000 patients. This patient had a history of excessive alcohol consumption prior to weight loss. He lost 150 pounds during the fasting phase of the program, and experienced foot drop during a drinking episode shortly after resumption of food intake. Improvement occurred within weeks.

CARDIAC ABNORMALITIES

The original report by Inser, describing 17 deaths in individuals who took liquid protein formula diet, created a stir in the medical community [9]. Eleven of these individuals had electrocardiographic evidence of ventricular tachycardia. Most had prolonged QT intervals on their electrocardiogram; and autopsy in some cases demonstrated myocardial atrophy. As a result the Federal Drug Administration withdrew the liquid protein formula diet from commercial use. Since then several perspective studies have been carried out on the effect of hypocaloric protein diets on cardiac function. Latingua conducted a 40 day study in 6 people who were given PROFAST, a protein formula of low biological value [10]. Three of the six individuals showed no electrocardiographic abnormalities by

Holter monitoring. A fourth patient developed second degree heart block and premature ventricular contractions; a fifth patient developed ventricular tachycardia; and a sixth sustained ventricular bigeminy. Shalom studied 13 patients who took OPTIFAST, a commercial protein formula composed of egg whites and sucrose, for 4, 8, and 12 weeks, respectively [11]. Neither arrythmia, low ARS voltage, nor prolongation of the QT interval was observed on the electrocardiogram in their 13 patients.

MORTALITY

Mortality data for subjects using a medically supervised PSMF, employing a high biological value protein, seem to indicate that it is a relatively safe procedure. Genuth et al. treated 2000 patients with such a PSMF and reported only six deaths [12]. Three of the fatalities had a prior history of coronary artery disease; one of the deaths was unexplained; one was accidental; and one was due to subacute bacterial endocarditis. In an attempt to reduce these risks our program at Wayne State University provides a thorough preprogram physical examination as well as weekly physical assessments for those in the PSMF program. To insure compliance with the PSMF protocol, participants are required to keep weekly records indicating when protein supplements were taken. The death rate associated with PSMF (less than 1 per 1000 individuals) compares favorably with an expected death rate of 3 for 104 from gastric bypass surgery [13].

ATTRITION

Attrition from treatment programs has been a consistent problem in the treatment of obesity. Figure 1 describes the percentage of patients remaining in different treatment programs after 12 weeks. Volkmar, Stunkard, Woolston, and Bailey examined five commercial weight reduction programs in three

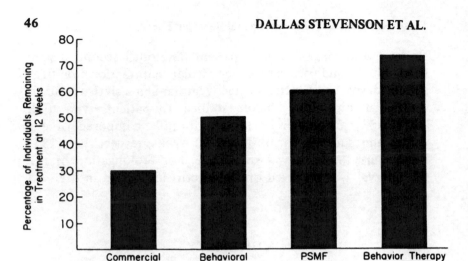

Figure 1. Percentage of patients remaining in treatment after 12 weeks.

different countries, and reported very similar attrition rates across different programs [14]. While 50% of participants remained in treatment for six weeks, only 30% remained by the twelfth week. Marston, Marston, and Ross had a much lower attrition rate in a behavioral correspondence course for weight reduction (50% of the population remaining by the twelfth week of treatment) [15]. Vertes and Hazelton used a combination of PSMF and weekly group sessions consisting of nutrition education, exercise training, and family orientation [12]. In their program 60% of the patients remained in treatment by the twelfth week. In our program, which also used PSMF in conjunction with weekly group therapy, 73% of patients remained in the program by the twelfth week. Thus, both PSMF treatment programs had fewer drop-outs than most treatments for obesity. This may be related to (a) the reinforcements associated with the rapid weight loss on PSMF, (b) selection variables associated with patients who choose this treatment, and (c) as yet undetermined variables. Nevertheless, there is a small but notable difference in

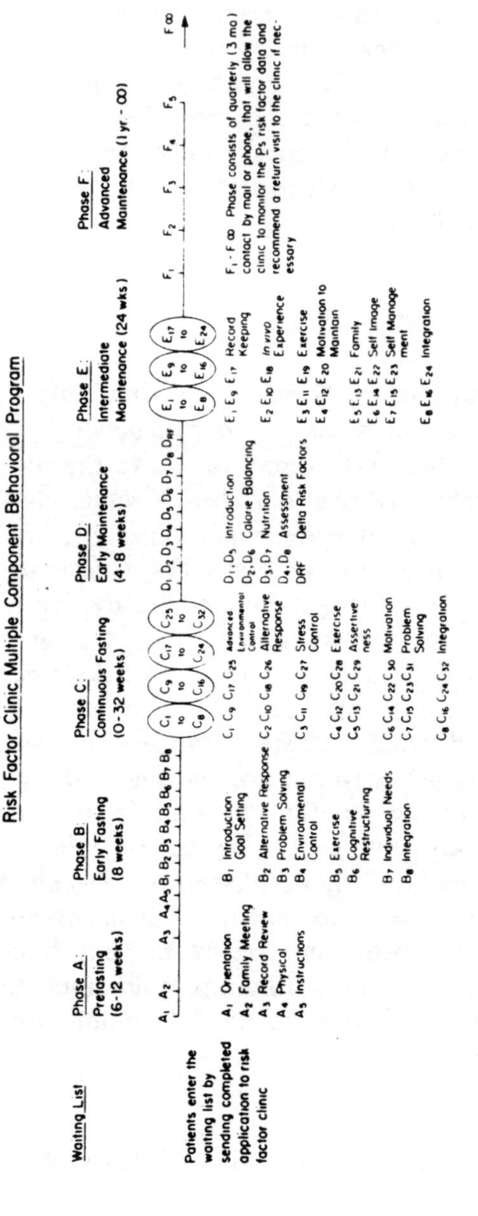

(Stevenson, Holmes and Ardito 1981)

Figure 2. The course of treatment for patients in the Wayne State University Risk Factor Program.

drop out rates between what was reported by Vertes et al. and the Wayne State University program. This is not inconsistent with Stunkard and Penick's finding that behavior therapy programs have less attrition than programs using only nutrition education [16]. Future work incorporating response cost or reinforcement system techniques similar to those used by Marston et al. may further reduce attrition of conjunctive PSMF behavioral treatment [15].

BEHAVIOR THERAPY

Behavior therapy in the Wayne State University program is presently conducted in weekly group sessions by a trained behavior analyst. There are several phases to the program (see Figure 2): *Prefasting* (Phase A), during which patients are taught how to self monitor exercise and consumptitory behavior. Meetings are held in groups with families, similar to Brownell [17] to prepare both the patient and family for the fasting phase of the program. *Fasting* (Phases B and C), where therapy focuses on teaching self analysis and control skills necessary to maintain compliance to the fast; and further prepares the patient for the maintenance phase of the program. *Maintenance* (Phases D, E, and F), devoted to teaching patterns of consumption and exercise compatible with the desired weight..Data is collected weekly by psychologists on target behaviors associated with each of these phases. At weekly meetings, clinic professionals meet to examine data, discuss patient strengths and weaknesses, and review current trends in the obesity literature. Through continuous evaluation the program is then modified to improve successful completion of these target behaviors.

AMOUNT AND RATE OF WEIGHT LOSS

There are many goals (reduction of risk factors, increased mobility, improved psychological functioning to name a few) in

the treatment of obesity. Most programs report results in terms
of weight reduction. It is very difficult to compare inter-pro-
gram data based on weight loss since individual patients have
different weight loss goals. Patient size also affects rate of loss
[1]. Therefore, even though several studies have reported
impressive average weekly weight losses (approximately 5
pounds per week) for programs employing a PSMF, it is difficult to evaluate success using this criterion [3, 18]. A more
useful method for measuring the success of an obesity program
would be to examine the approximation to "ideal weight"
(given the lack of evidence for the notion of ideal weight, the
term reference weight will be used) achieved by every individual
who enters treatment. In order to examine the effectiveness of
the Wayne State University program, data was collected on each
person (N = 267) who entered the program during a six month
period. Figure 3 shows where individuals fell on a scale between

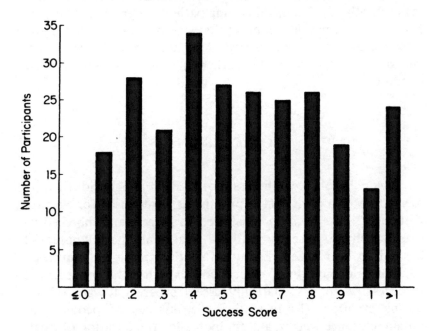

Figure 3. Number of participants within each success score category
(total N = 267).

0 (no success) and 1 (total success). This success scale only demonstrates approximations to reference weight. Future scales may include other important treatment targets. This number was determined by dividing weight loss (starting weight minus weight at last visit) by starting weight minus reference weight (upper limit of Metropolitan tables). Using this criterion, 14% achieved reference weight, and approximately 60% were able to lose half the weight they needed to lose. Average weight loss equalled 56 pounds per person. In conclusion, the combination of PSMF and behavioral treatment, as practiced in the Wayne State University program is more effective in terms of lower attrition and average weight loss than most other therapies presently available. (More useful comparisons could be made if future researchers would report results in terms of approximation to reference weight). Important components of the program include experienced professionals (physicians, behavior analysts, nurses, and office staff) continuously interacting with (a) each other, (b) data describing patient progress, and (c) professional literature, in a context that supports evolution of more effective treatments for obesity. Generalizations of these results will occur to the extent that other facilities can recreate these conditions.

CONCLUSION

In conclusion, a combination of PSMF and behavior therapy seems to hold a great deal of promise as a treatment for obesity. Although it has been demonstrated to be safe and more effective than many presently available treatments, its full potential has yet to be realized. Evolution of this treatment requires a continued integration of clinical and experimental processes. It is necessary to systematically assess progress toward (a) reducing attrition, (b) increasing the number of people who obtain reference weight, and (c) increasing the duration of treatment results.

ACKNOWLEDGEMENT

We gratefully acknowledge the assistance of Pat Hinton for her effort in completing the statistical analysis. We would also like to thank Cheryl Duffy and Diane Snapp for typing the manuscript.

REFERENCES

1. Stunkard, A. J. Behavioral treatment of obesity: the current status. *Int. J. Obesity 2*:237, 1977.
2. Genuth, S. M., Vertes, V., and Castro, J. H. Weight reduction in obesity by outpatient semistarvation. *Am. Med. Assoc. 230*:987, 1974.
3. Blackburn, G. L., Sizer, J. S., Bistrian, B. R., and Rogers, J. F. Effects of modified starvation on balke performance in well trained subjects. *Clin. Res. 24*:357A, 1976.
4. Apfelbaum, M., Boudon, P., Nillus, P., and Lacatis, D. Effects metaboliques de la diete protidique chez 41 subjects obeses. *Presse Med. 78*: 1917, 1970.
5. Genuth, S. Supplemented fasting in the treatment of obesity and diabetes. *The Am. J. Clin. Nutr. 32*:2579, 1979.
6. Marliss, E. B., Murray, F. T., and Nakhooda, A. F. The metabolic response to hypocaloric protein diets in obese man. *J. Clin. Invest. 62*:468, 1978.
7. Bistrian, B. R., Blackburn, D. L., Flatt, J. P., Sizer, J., Scrimshaw, N., and Sherman, M. Nitrogen metabolism and insulin requirements in obese diabetic adults on a protein-sparing modified fast. *Diabetes 25*:494, 1976.
8. Fisler, J. S., Drenick, R. J., Blumfield, D. E., and Swengeid, M. D. Nitrogen economy during very low calorie reducing diets: quality and quantity of dietary protein. *The Am. J. Clin. Nutr. 35*:471, 1982.
9. Isner, J. M., Sours, J. E., Paris, A. L., Ferrans, V. J., and Roberts, W. C. Sudden unexpected death in avid dieters using the liquid protein-modified fast diet: observations in 17 patients and the role of the prolonged QT interval. *Circulation 60*:1401, 1979.

10. Lantigua, R. A., Amatruda, N. M., Biddle, T. L., Forbes, G. B., and Lockwood, D. H. Cardiac arrhythmias associated with a liquid protein diet for the treatment of obesity. *N. Eng. J. Med. 303*:735, 1980.

11. Shalom, R. M., Santora, L. J., Meltzer, P., Horovitz, E., and Henry, W. L. Ventricular ectopy in markedly obese subjects before and after rapid weight loss. *American Heart Association's 54th Scientific Sessions*, Dallas, Texas, November 1981.

12. Genuth, S. M., Vertes, V., and Hazelton, I. Supplemented fasting in the treatment of obesity. *Rec. Adv. Ob. Resrch. 2*:370, 1979.

13. Murphy, K., McCracken, J. D., and Ozment, K. L. Gastric bypass for obesity. *Am. Surg. 140*:747, 1980.

14. Volkmar, R. R., Stunkard, A. J., Woolston, J., and Bailey, R. A. High attrition rates in commercial weight reduction program. *Arch. Intern. Med. 141*:426, 1981.

15. Marston, A. R., Marston, M. R., and Ross, J. A correspondence course behavioral program for weight reduction. *Obesity Bariatric Med. 6*: 4, 1977.

16. Stunkard, A. J., and Penick, S. B. Behavior modification in the treatment of obesity: The problem of maintaining weight loss. *Arch. Gen. Psychiatry 36*:801, 1979.

17. Kirschner, M. A., et al. Supplemented starvation: a successful method for control of major obesity. *J. Med. Soc. N.J. 76*:175, 1979.

18. Brownell, K. The effect of spouse training and partner cooperativeness in the behavioral treatment of obesity. Unpublished doctoral dissertation, Rutgers University, 1978.

4

Myths and Misconceptions in Exercise for Weight Control

Barry A. Franklin

INTRODUCTION

Over the past 20 years considerable research has focused on the effectiveness of various intervention strategies in the treatment of obesity. Caloric restriction (energy intake) rather than physical activity (energy expenditure) manipulations have received the greatest attention. One comprehensive review reported that physical activity was examined in only 6% of all weight control studies [1].

Recently, exercise has been proposed as a viable alternative or adjunct to the dietary treatment of obesity [2]. This shift in attention has resulted primarily from two lines of experimental evidence: Studies evaluating the efficacy of dietary intervention on weight reduction have generally shown minimal results with poor long-term compliance. Some research suggests that physiologic mechanisms (i.e., the body's adaptive lowering of the basal metabolic rate during food deprivation) may counteract the effect of dieting [3].

With the popularity of exercise increasing, obese individuals are oftentimes confronted with exercise myths and misconceptions, along with gadgets and gimmicks that are promoted as "miracle agents" to assist in weight reduction. Although some of these are beneficial and effective, many have no practical value.

The purposes of this paper are (1) to review the physiologic basis of exercise training in weight reduction programs; (2) to clarify many of the myths and misconceptions regarding the role of exercise in reducing body weight and fat stores, with reference to active versus passive exercise devices; and (3) to highlight the optimal exercise prescription for overweight therapy.

CALORIC COST OF EXERCISE

The effectiveness of exercise in the control of body weight has been minimized by many who claim that the amount of activity required to significantly affect caloric output is prohibitive [4]. The rationale behind this logic undoubtedly stems from energy equivalent tables that present the rate of caloric expenditure for various physical activities. Comparison of these rates with the energy expenditure necessary to burn one pound of fat often leads to discouragement among those who would like to reduce body weight through exercise.

Exercise proponents feel the "misconception" that exercise requires little caloric expenditure can be discounted by noting that laborers, soldiers in the field, and endurance athletes can consume some 6,000 calories (kcal) daily, yet remain thin. Such excessive caloric intakes contradict the belief that physical activity plays a negligable role in energy balance.

On the other hand, exercise critics present data that illustrate the need for thirty-six hours of walking, eleven hours of volleyball, seven hours of chopping wood—or some other ridiculous amount of physical activity—to lose one pound of weight. These extremes of muscular exercise discredit the possibility of reducing weight by increased physical activity, since they imply that the exercise must be done at one time. Exercise enthusiasts argue that the "cumulative caloric expenditure" is of major importance and suggest that an increase in gross energy expenditure of only 75 to 100 kcal per day (approximately equal to walking one mile per day for most persons), with caloric intake unchanged, will result in a 10 pound weight loss per year [5]. Others [3,6] however, suggest that this logic is misleading, that the true caloric effect of exercise must consider the net energy cost of the exercise bout, this calculated as the total energy cost of the exercise minus the energy cost of normal activity during the same time period. For most individuals the net cost of exercise is approximately two kcal per minute less than the gross cost [7]. Thus, if an individual walks 30 minutes and expends 150 kcal, the net cost of the exercise is 90 kcal, not 150 kcal.

Since a pound of weight is lost with a negative caloric balance of approximately 3,500 kcal, it is apparent that if only net energy expenditure is considered, a substantial amount of exercise is required to facilitate a significant weight loss. Fortunately the caloric expenditure associated with exercise is not limited to the time of the activity alone.

Metabolic After Effects of Exercise

It is well documented that in the postexercise recovery period more oxygen is consumed than is required to sustain resting metabolism; this phenomenon is known as recovery oxygen debt [8,9]. Delayed postexercise return of oxygen consumption to resting levels has been attributed to numerous factors including the conversion of lactate to glucose and adenosine triphosphate, augmented cardiopulmonary metabolism, increased body temperature, elevated catecholamine levels, and, more recently, "substrate cycling" [10].

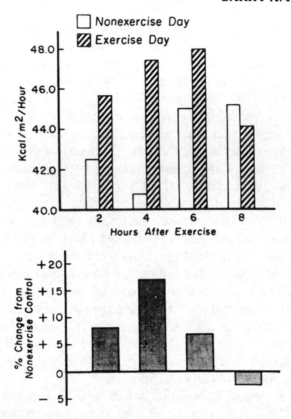

Figure 1. Top: Resting metabolic rate, expressed as kcal/m^2/hour, after a vigorous exercise session compared with a nonexercise control day. Bottom: Resting metabolic rate was from 6% to 17% higher after a vigorous exercise session than it was at the same time of day on nonexercise control days. Furthermore, the higher metabolic rate was shown to persist at least six hours after exercise. Adapted from de Vries and Gray [14].

As long ago as 1933, Edwards and associates [9,11] demonstrated an increased resting metabolic rate that lasted for several hours after cessation of vigorous exercise, 10% and 25% above basal for as long as 48 and 15 hours, respectively. Recent analyses of these data suggest that strenuous exercise may produce an additional expenditure of 450 kcal subsequent to the cessation of physical activity [12]. Others, however, have demonstrated less dramatic increases in postexercise metabolism. For example, Passmore and Johnson [13] found that oxygen consumption remained 14% to 18% higher than normal for 7 hours after workout.

The most systematic study of the metabolic aftereffects of exercise was performed by de Vries and Gray [14]. Results indicated that the resting metabolic rate ranged from 7.5% to 28% higher 4 hours after exercise compared with a control day in which no exercise was taken. This higher metabolic rate persisted for 6 hours and returned to baseline levels after 8 hours (Figure 1). The investigators calculated that this elevated postexercise metabolism, over and above the energy cost of the exercise bout itself, approximated 40 to 50 kcal, and would have resulted in the caloric equivalent of four or five pounds per year if the individuals tested had exercised daily.

In summary, it appears that exercise is beneficial in the control of body weight, not only for the energy losses incurred during the exercise but also because a considerable additional caloric expenditure may occur following exercise. Clearly, additional research is needed to test various activities at differing intensities and durations to determine the optimal exercise regimen to induce prolonged elevation of the postexercise metabolic rate.

EXERCISE AND APPETITE

One misconception that has been cited to frequently discount the benefits of exercise in weight control is the contention that physical activity always stimulates the appetite and increases caloric intake, negating the caloric expenditure of the exercise itself [4,5]. Although it is true that an increase in food intake generally parallels an increase in physical activity, research has shown that this relationship appears to hold only within a certain activity zone, i.e., normal activity.

Mayer and associates demonstrated that at extremely high or low levels of daily energy expenditure appetite no longer worked as a guide to balancing food intake and energy

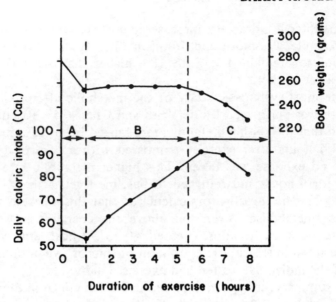

Figure 2. Relationship between food intake, energy expenditure, and body weight in laboratory rats. A = sedentary zone; B = range of proportional response (normal activity); C = exhaustion zone. Adapted from Mayer [15].

expenditure [15,16]. For example, rats exercised daily for up to one hour showed a decrease in food intake and body weight when compared to sedentary control animals [15]. When the exercise duration was increased beyond one hour, food intake increased, but only to the extent that body weight was maintained. In contrast, at exhaustive levels of exercise (i.e., 6 hours), both body weight and food intake decreased. Figure 2 illustrates the results of this classic experiment [15].

A nonlinear relation between caloric intake and energy expenditure has also been demonstrated in humans (Figure 3). Mayer and associates [16] measured caloric intake and physical activity in an industrial population in which five occupational activity categories (from sedentary to very heavy work) were established. The results substantiated their earlier findings [15] in animals illustrating a linear relationship between activity level and caloric intake, but only within the light-to-heavy activity range. Again, those in the sedentary range tended to weigh more

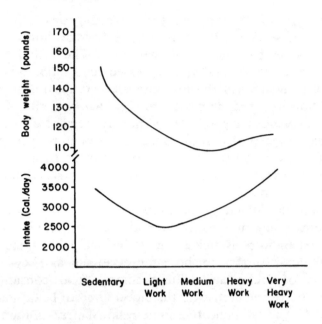

Figure 3. Body weight and caloric intake as related to occupational physical activity in humans. Adapted from Mayer [16].

and consume a greater number of calories than did those who engaged in light-to-medium activity.

From his studies in animals and man, Mayer has concluded that when physical activity is reduced below a minimum level, a corresponding decrease in food intake does not result and obesity develops [4,5]. He has referred to this activity level as the sedentary or "non-responsive zone," in view of the nonlinear relationship between caloric intake and energy expenditure [15]. Such knowledge has long been empirically employed by farmers who confine or "pen-up" cattle and hogs for fattening [5].

Longitudinal physical conditioning studies in humans have generally shown no change in caloric intake with mild to moderate intensity exercise training [17–21]. In contrast, vigorous exercise of short duration has been shown to decrease appetite in male rats [22–24]. These findings prompted the suggestion that appetite suppression may depend on the intensity and duration of the exercise [25]. Testing this hypothesis, Katch and co-workers [26] studied the effects of short duration caloric cost in two groups of male rats. The high intensity exercise group demonstrated a depressed food intake and body weight gain relative to the low intensity group. Both exercise groups, however, had depressed food intake and rate of body weight increase compared to nonexercise control animals. These data suggest that short bouts of strenuous exercise are more effective in decreasing food consumption than moderate exercise of extended duration. However, similar findings in humans are lacking.

Several physiologic mechanisms have been cited to explain how exercise may suppress or maintain at a constant level while energy expenditure is increasing. Baile and co-workers [27] reported food intake to be suppressed in monkeys given injections of lactic acid. Furthermore, food consumption remained decreased even after the blood levels of lactic acid had returned to normal, indicating some residual effect. Others have suggested that appetite suppression or maintenance following exercise may be mediated by increases in plasma catecholamines [24,25], increases in core temperature [28], or the formation of "anorexigenic substances" [29].

WALKING VS. RUNNING VS. OUTDOOR BICYCLING: COMPARISON OF CALORIC EXPENDITURE

Activities frequently employed in weight reduction and cardiovascular fitness programs include running, walking, and outdoor bicycling. However, in spite of the considerable data available regarding the energy cost of these exercise modes, there seems to be disagreement as to the number of kcal expended per unit distance for each activity.

The caloric cost of walking versus running a given distance has been the subject of considerable controversy. It is claimed that the longer exercise duration involved in walking a given distance results in approximately the same caloric expenditure as running that same distance over a shorter period of time [30].

The laws of physics would appear to confirm this hypothesis, in that a given weight moves a given distance by both methods.

On the other hand, previous research [31–34] and recent well-designed studies [35–36] indicate that running a given distance expends more kcal than walking the same distance, whether the energy cost is expressed or an absolute or net basis (total energy expenditure minus resting energy expenditure over the entire duration). These findings are also compatible with the American College of Sports Medicine energy cost calculations for walking and running [37].

Our review of the literature suggests that the gross caloric cost of walking and running is approximately 1.15 and 1.70 kcal/kg/mile, respectively (Figure 4) [38]. Furthermore, unless the walking or running speed is extremely fast or slow for each method, the caloric cost per unit distance is relatively independent of speed. For example, walking at 2.0 and 4.0 mph requires 1.35 and 1.20 kcal/kg/mile, respectively, equivalent to 95 and 84 kcal per mile for a 70 kg man [39]. Running at 6.0 and 10.0 mph requires 1.60 and 1.80 kcal/kg/mile, respectively, equivalent to 112 and 126 kcal per mile for a 70 kg man [39].

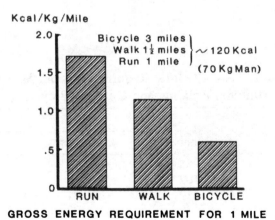

Figure 4. Gross caloric cost per mile for running, walking, and outdoor bicycling. For each of the exercise modes the caloric cost per unit distance is relatively independent of speed. Adapted from Franklin and Rubenfire [38].

These data imply that the particular walking or running speed, when within the normal range, has little effect on the total energy expenditure, expressed per unit distance. Although many overweight persons may be unable to run, a substantial energy expenditure can result from walking a longer distance.

Outdoor bicycling is an energy-efficient method of covering distance. Although the energy cost of bicycle riding varies with the type of bicycle, cycling skill of the individual, and body weight, the gross caloric cost approximates 0.60 kcal/kg/mile [38]. Like walking and running, the caloric cost per unit distance is also relatively independent of speed. For example, bicycling at 5.0 and 13.0 mph requires 0.60 and 0.75 kcal/kg/ mile, respectively, equivalent to 42 and 53 kcal per mile for a 70 kg man [39]. For a given distance, one uses approximately one half the kcal of brisk walking and one third the kcal of running if you bicycle it. Expressed another way, the energy cost of bicycling 3 miles is the approximate equivalent of walking 1.5 miles or running 1.0 mile (Figure 4) [38]. Table 1 provides a comparison of the gross caloric expenditure per mile for walking, running, and outdoor cycling as a function of body weight.

Table 1.   Gross Caloric Requirements per Mile for
Running, Walking, and Outdoor Bicycling

Body weight		kcal/mile		
(lbs)	(kg)	Running	Walking	Bicycling
110	50	85	58	30
132	60	102	69	36
154	70	119	81	42
176	80	136	92	48
198	90	153	104	54
220	100	170	115	60
242	110	187	127	66
264	120	204	138	72

Adapted from Franklin and Rubenfire [38].

EFFORTLESS WEIGHT REDUCTION

Mechanical Vibrators

Passive exercise gadgets that "do the work for you" have been touted as effortless exercise devices that take off or redistribute body fat. Several years ago Hernlund and Steinhaus [40] investigated the validity of the weight-reducing claims made for the mechanical vibrating machines commonly used in health clubs and gymnasiums (Figure 5). The investigators hypothesized that if the device oxidized or "massaged away" body fat, somatic oxygen uptake and/or blood fats should be increased.

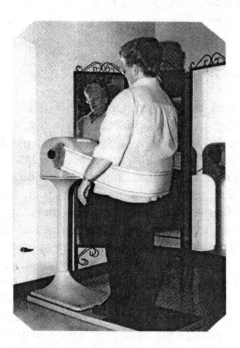

Figure 5. A woman leans back against a vibrator belt, hoping its massage will reduce body weight and fat stores.

Thirteen men, some considerably overweight, were subjected to a 15-minute period of continuous abdominal vibration. During and after the "exercise bout" measures of oxygen consumption (for caloric cost) were made. In addition, venous blood fats were drawn before and shortly after exercise, and again two or three hours later.

Results of the study revealed that blood fats remained essentially unchanged from the pre-exercise control period. Average caloric cost of the 15-minute exercise session, including recovery, was 11.4 kcal more than each man would have expended had he remained seated at rest for an equivalent period of time. This "net cost" represents approximately 1/19th of an ounce of fat. Thus, to lose a pound of fat (3,500 kcal) would have required 307 such 15-minute periods of abdominal vibration, or roughly six exercise sessions per week for a year!

The investigators concluded that "the vibrator is not to be taken seriously as a device to assist in fat reduction or shifting of fat deposits within the body."

Passive Exercise Devices

Over the past twenty years a variety of effortless exercise devices including roller machines (Figures 6 and 7), oscillating tables, massagers, electrically driven stationary bicycles, and similar laborsaving equipment, have been introduced as "easy ways" to improve the figure and reduce body weight [41]. "Active physical exercise improves your figure—trims you, makes you firmer—makes you look slimmer and more attractive," said a brochure from the manufacturer of Relax-A-Cizor, a low-voltage electrical muscle-stimulating apparatus. "But how tiresome it is! If you have ever tried 'exercises' you must often have said to yourself, 'There must be an easier way!' And now there is! At last . . . Effortless Beautifying Exercise!"

Approximately 350,000 Relax-A-Cizor devices were sold at up to $350 each [41]. Although the manufacturer never claimed the device could take off weight, the gadget was promoted as "an easy way to improve your figure." However,

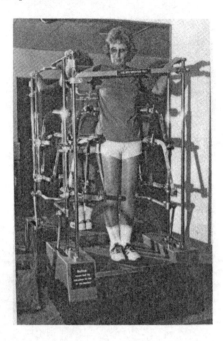

Figure 6. Electrically-powered ring roller exercise device provides simultaneous massage to the leg, hip, stomach, and back areas.

according to The Food and Drug Administration, "There is no device which will be effective for 'spot reducing,' for 'melting away fat,' of for 'breaking up fatty deposits.'" Another example, the "Magic Couch," promoted by its manufacturer as an effortless exercise device to lose weight, was reported by the Federal Trade Commission to be "of no value in reducing weight."

Effortless exercise devices are, at best, capable only of moving fatty tissue, not removing it. The potential for exercise to contribute to a negative caloric balance and body fat loss is illustrated by the physical laws that govern net energy exchange, most simply expressed as:

Caloric balance = kilocalories from food – (kilocalories of basal metabolism + kilocalories of exercise metabolism + kilocalories lost in excreta)

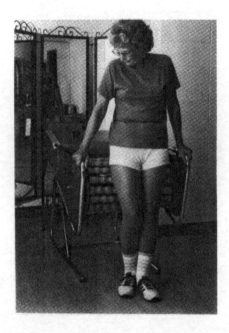

Figure 7. Operation of the electrically-powered Roaler Massager exercise device.

It is apparent that exercise can influence caloric balance, but only in direct proportion to the amount of human effort expressed as kilocalories expended. " 'Effortless exercise,' " according to Dr. Gordon M. Martin, "is certainly nothing but a high-sounding phrase that is about as meaningful as 'foodless meal' " [41].

Weight Reducing Clothing

Special weight-reducing clothing, including heated belts, rubberized suits, and oilskins, are semipermeable or impermeable to sweat and rely chiefly on dehydration (removal of body water), localized pressure, or tissue compression [38]. Although circumference measures or scale weight may temporarily decrease, these losses are unrelated to reductions in body fat.

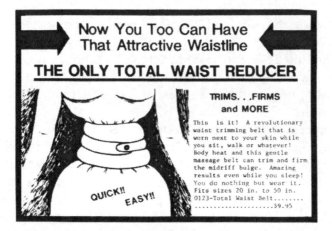

Figure 8. Typical waist-belt advertisement often found in health, fashion and women's magazines.

Heat or pressurized waist belts serve to drive water out of localized tissue areas. Circumference or tape measures may be temporarily reduced until rehydration occurs. Clever advertisers prey on this fact to highlight the benefits of their product which can reduce the waist, "even while sleeping." A typical waist-belt advertisement, often found in health-fitness, fashion, or women's magazines, is shown in Figure 8.

Impermeable or semipermeable exercise clothing acts to increase water losses and dangerously restricts evaporative cooling. A greater-than-normal loss of water, not fat, results. This dehydration causes a reduction in effective circulating blood volume and a subsequent drop in blood pressure. As a result, heart rate increases disproportionately to keep up with increasing metabolic demands [42].

Oilskins and rubberized sweat suits worn during exercise are potentially dangerous since they block convective heat loss and the evaporation of sweat, thus depriving the body of its normal mechanism for cooling. It is important to note that it is the evaporation of sweat, rather than sweating per se, that serves as the major mechanism for heat dissipation during vigorous exercise. With impermeable clothing, the heat and sweat given off between the suit and the skin remain trapped. Trapped sweat can't evaporate to cool the body, and convective heat loss is also inhibited. The increased exercise metabolic rate, coupled with the added burden imposed on the temperature regulating mechanism, may result in a severe rise in core temperature and heat disorders.

An excessive loss of body water is useless for weight control and may be dangerous. Depleted body water is rapidly replenished with food and liquid consumption. Body weight (fat) is lost only when caloric expenditure, including the calories used in basal metabolism and physical activity, exceed the caloric intake. Water contains no calories! Thus, special weight reducing clothing is not only ineffective but potentially dangerous, since it may intensify the heat load on the body.

Ideally, the most effective clothing for reduction of body fat is clothing that promotes energy expenditure and/or caloric restriction. Unfortunately, no material has yet been fabricated that effects these lifestyle changes. It is not suprising that some manufacturers have included in their advertising (in small print, of course) the recommendation that a diet or fitness program accompany wearing of their "incredible" weight reducing garment to maximize effectiveness [38].

ACTIVE EXERCISE DEVICES: A CRITIQUE

Bust Developers

Numerous exercise devices and programs are advertised to increase bust size. Recently, Wilmore and co-workers [43] investigated the effectiveness of one of the best known programs, the 21-day Mark Eden "Mark II" bust developer program. Thirty-four women, 19 to 32 years of age, were randomly assigned to either control or experimental groups to assess alterations in breast size, shape, and volume using the Mark Eden exercise device as recommended by the manufacturer. Exercise and control groups were evaluated twice before initiating the bust developing program to establish reliability of the test procedures and again at the program conclusion. Pre-post training evaluations included bust girths with and without bra, front and side view breast photography, both jn the full inspiration and full expiration position, and measures of breast volume, using a water displacement technique. Results indicated no significant difference in bust girth or breast volume consequent to the program. It was concluded that the Mark Eden "Mark II" Bust Developer Program does not alter breast size, shape, or volume.

Rebound Exercise

Rebound exercise devices, relatively new to the fitness scene, are promoted as the optimal means to "trauma-reduced aerobic exercise." The units resemble minitrampolines, except the bouncing area is larger (Figure 9). By design the jumping surface

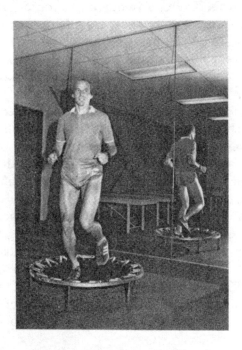

Figure 9. Rebound running units are relatively new to the fitness scene.

is level rather than tilted, to prevent the acrobatics that are possible on minitrampolines.

Manufacturers claim that rebounders reduce stress on the ankles, knees, and legs that often results from running on hard surfaces. Unfortunately, some previous advertising used by rebounding service representatives and distributors has been misleading and unfounded, with miraculous beneficial claims for a variety of ailments [44].

Until recently, few data were available regarding the physiologic adaptation to regular rebound training, particularly as it compares to conventional conditioning modes. The first published study on rebounding investigated whether rebounding was as effective in improving fitness and reducing body fat as running or stationary cycle ergometry [45]. Three groups of overweight women exercised a 10-week period. One group trained with treadmill exercise, another used stationary cycle ergometry, the third, rebounding. Ten overweight women served as controls. Exercise frequency, duration, and intensity for each group were 4 days/week, 30 minutes per session, at an average heart rate of 150 beats/minute. Aerobic capacity (VO_2 max) and percent body fatness were measured before and after the training program (Table 2). All groups showed similar improvements in VO_2 max and decrements in percent body fatness, while control subjects remained unchanged. It was concluded that rebounding is comparable to treadmill running and stationary cycle ergometry in increasing fitness or decreasing body fat in overweight women. These results, however, have been criticized since several of the women were simultaneously dieting during the study period [44].

Katch and co-workers [46] examined the energy cost and heart rate response of rebound running among healthy but sedentary young-to-middle-aged subjects. Results showed an average heart rate and oxygen consumption of 116 beats/minute and 17ml/ kg/min, respectively. These data indicate that rebound running requires an average intensity of 5 times the resting metabolic rate (5 METS), representing a low-to-moderate

Table 2. Effect of Rebound Training, Treadmill Exercise,
and Stationary Cycle Ergometry on Aerobic Capacity
and Percent Body Fatness in Overweight Women

Variable	Group	Training		Δ
		Pre	Post	
VO_2 max, ml/kg/min	Rebound	30.4	33.9	+3.5
	Treadmill	31.8	35.5	+3.7
	Cycle	30.5	33.8	+3.3
Percent body fat	Rebound	31.2	27.2	-4.0
	Treadmill	31.3	26.4	-4.9
	Cycle	30.9	28.3	-2.6

Adapted from White [45].

intensity activity, equivalent to walking at approximately a 4.0 mph pace. However, many subjects were unable to significantly increase the stepping rate while maintaining normal rebound height. As a result, few individuals were able to attain relatively high exercise heart rates. Others have also experienced this restriction [47]. In addition, the energy cost of rebound running has been shown to be considerably below that required to run on a treadmill at the same heart rate [44], a limitation previously reported for skipping rope [48].

In summary, the verdict on rebound running is still out. Additional scientific data are needed. It appears that some of the claims made by the manufacturers of rebounders should be viewed with caution. Rebounding may be a reasonable way to improve physical fitness and decrease body fat, particularly among sedentary adults initiating exercise programs [47]. Although it may also aid in reducing musculoskeletal and orthopedic problems associated with conventional exercise programs, it appears that intensity limitations of "standard rebound running" may limit it's effectiveness as a cardiovascular conditioner and weight reduction apparatus.

SPOT REDUCTION

The concept of "spot reduction" is based on the widely held belief that it is possible to selectively "burn off" fat from a particular part of the body by exercising that body area. Indeed spot reducing programs have become a multi-million dollar industry in a country where the health and aesthetic disadvantages of excessive adiposity are well-recognized.

Considerable research, summarized by an excellent recent review [49], casts considerable doubt on the concept of spot reduction. Although Olson and Edelstein [50] concluded that vigorous exercise of a specific body area will result in a reduction of subcutaneous tissue in that area, most scientific data suggests that spot reduction techniques are ineffective. Carns and associates [51] reported no difference in generalized versus localized exercise programs on segmental volume among women who participated in these exercise regimens. Roby [52] investigated the effect of weight training on the triceps skinfold thickness of a regularly exercised and nonexercised control arm. Skinfolds decreased equally over the exercised and nonexercised triceps, refuting the postulate that subcutaneous fat is disproportionately reduced in the specific region where muscles are exercised. Finally, Schade and co-workers [53] reported no significant difference in the effect of spot and generalized exercise on fat reduction, a position generally supported by a recent review of the subject [49].

Gwinup and associates [54] evaluated the validity of the concept of spot reduction by comparing the circumference and subcutaneous fat of the active (playing) and inactive arm of accomplished tennis players. It was hypothesized that if exercise of a particular body part selectively reduced fat tissue in that area, then the racquet or playing arm should have considerably less fat than the inactive arm. Although circumference measures in the active (playing) arm were greater than the nonplaying arm due to muscular hypertrophy, skinfold thickness measures revealed no difference in subcutaneous fat deposits between the arms. The investigators concluded that these data provide direct evidence against the concept of spot reduction.

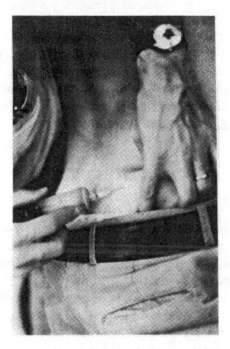

Figure 10. Fat biopsy sampling technique. (Photo courtesy of Dr. Frank Katch).

Perhaps the most convincing evidence against spot reduction comes from recent studies of the effects of localized abdominal exercise training on regional adipose cell size [55]. Abdominal, gluteal, and subscapular fat biopsies were taken from 15 experimental and 6 control subjects before and after a 27 day abdominal exercise training program (Figure 10). Progressive overload abdominal training was employed, 5 days/week, to a total of 5,000 sit-ups! Fat cell diameter decreased significantly at all three sampling sites, with no significant differences in the rate of change among sites. These data imply that localized exercise (i.e., sit-ups) do not preferentially reduce abdominal adipose cell size.

Although exercising muscle uses fatty acids as a primary energy source, particularly during mild-to-moderate-intensity exertion [56], there is presently no evidence to suggest that fatty acids diffuse into the muscle from its overlying fat pad. Instead, it appears that fatty acids from adipose tissue stores throughout the body are mobilized during exercise to supply the needed energy fuels. Perhaps one reason why spot reducing sometimes seems to work is that if the exercise intensity or duration is strenuous enough it will cause fat from the entire body (including a particular target area) to be reduced.

CELLULITE CURES

Cellulite is the term used to describe a unique and unsightly type of fatty tissue, causing the overlying skin to appear dimpled like an orange peel. It is believed to be different from normal fat in that if squeezed, the pinched tissue produces lumps and bulges. Proponents claim that trapped fat in the connective tissue, a major layer of the skin, is responsible for this distortion.

Although most medical and nutrition authorities contend that cellulite is simply subcutaneous fat of a different con-sistancy, the cosmetics industry insists that cellulite does exist. French cosmeticians describe it as a chronic inflammation of the connective tissue which "impedes the flow of blood and lymph." Supposedly, 80 percent of all women and 10 percent of men have cellulite deposits located primarily in the thigh, buttocks, and knee areas [57].

Several exercise and/or diet programs have been touted as "miracle cellulite cures." One well-known treatment regimen involves a high-protein diet, including large amounts of water and no salt. The diet is to be accompanied by massage of the cellulite areas to "break up connective tissue bridges and their adjacent fat stores." In addition, mild calisthenics are often recommended specifically for cellulite removal.

Although it is true that vigorous exercise and caloric re-striction will cause a general reduction in body fat stores, including localized fat deposits, there is no conclusive scientific evidence that high protein diets, massage, sauna, special skin creams, body wrappings, or pseudoelectric devices will break up or reduce cellulite deposits. Exorbitant fees are frequently charged for these unfounded cures. Unfortunately, the only reduction often occurs in the subscriber's wallet.

BODY COMPOSITION ALTERATIONS WITH EXERCISE TRAINING

Regular exercise training has a favorable effect on body composition, combating the trend toward adult onset obesity (increased fat cell size). A recent review [58] of longitudinal training studies in humans concluded that "exercise training appears to result in moderate losses of total body weight, moderate-to-large losses in body fat, and small-to-moderate increases in lean body weight." However, inspection of these compiled data reveals that the alterations in body composition with exercise training are small; for example, the average loss in percent body fatness across the studies cited was only 1.6%. Furthermore, many investigations showed slight decreases or unchanged lean body weight with physical conditioning, the variability perhaps attributed to concommitant caloric restriction in some cases.

Several years ago we studied the effects of a 12-week (4 day/week) physical conditioning program on the body composition of sedentary normal weight and obese middle-aged women [59]. Thirty-six premenopausal women (age range 29–47 years), i.e., 23 obese (>30% body fatness, $\bar{x} = 38\%$) and 13 lean to normal women (<30% body fatness, $\bar{x} = 25\%$), served as subjects. The exercise program included a 10-minute calisthenic warm-up, 15 to 25 minutes of walking–jogging at an individually prescribed training heart rate corresponding to 75% of maximal oxygen uptake, modified recreational games involving sustained total body movement (Figure 11), and a 5-minute cool-down. Body composition changes calculated from body density determined by hydrostatic weighing (Figure 12) are shown in Table 3. Body weight and fatness decreased slightly in the lean to normal subjects, and more in the obese women, while fat-free weight remained unchanged in both groups.

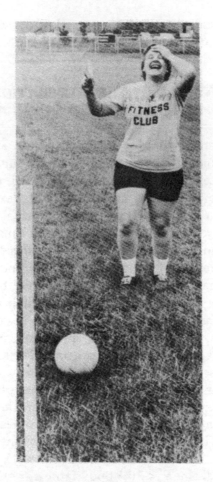

Figure 11. A "Franklin Fitness Club" participant plays a round of kick-ball golf. Rules are similar to conventional golf, except that soccer balls and wooden stakes (holes) are employed.

Stability in fat-free weight for both groups appears to contradict the generally held belief that physical conditioning always stimulates an enlargement of the musculature. Sexual differences in response do not represent a viable explanation since numerous studies in middle-aged men have also shown no change in fat-free weight following an exercise regimen

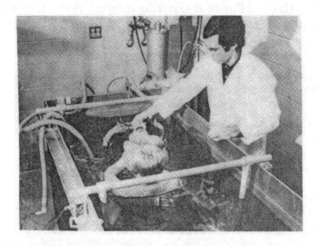

Figure 12. Underwater weighing system showing subject resting with her head out of water prior to initiation of weighing procedure. Equipment and methods are those of Akers and Buskirk [60].

[62–64]. In contrast, postconditioning increments in fat-free weight were reported in lean and obese young men [65] and obese adolescent women [66]. These data suggest that although younger persons may have a tendency to increase fat-free mass with physical conditioning, muscle mass is not appreciably increased in middle-aged subjects who participate in physical conditioning programs involving rhythmic, relatively low resistance exercise.

Our results also revealed that exercise-induced fat weight losses closely parallel ($r = 0.94$) those of total body weight. A high correlation between decreases in body fat and total body weight is consistent with previous data that suggests an increased fat loss/weight loss ratio when the energy deficit is achieved by increased exercise with or without caloric restriction as opposed to caloric restriction alone [67]. Estimates of the contribution of lean tissue to the total weight loss in response to caloric restriction alone have amounted to as much as 45 percent [61,68, 69]. Conservation of lean tissue may be due to increased fatty acid mobilization and utilization during

Table 3. Effect of Physical Conditioning on Body Composition
Calculated from Changes in Body Weight and Density
in Normal (N) and Obese (O) Women

Variable	Group	Pre	Post	Δ	P
Body weight,	N	54.16	53.76	-0.40	NS
kg	O	75.97	73.41	-2.56	<.001
Density[a]	N	1.041	1.043	+0.002	<.05
gm/cc	O	1.011	1.015	+0.004	<.001
Percent body fat[b]	N	24.7	23.9	-0.8	<.05
	O	38.0	36.2	-1.8	<.001
Fat-free body	N	40.78	40.90	+0.12	NS
weight, kg	O	46.91	46.63	-0.28	NS
Fat weight,	N	13.38	12.86	-0.52	<.05
kg	O	29.06	26.78	-2.28	<.001

Adapted from Franklin et al. [59]
[a]Density calculated according to the underwater weighing procedure of
Akers and Buskirk [60].
[b]Percent body fat calculated from body density by the method of Brozek
et al. [61], where percent fat = $100 [(4.570/D_b) - 4.142]$

and after exercise [70,71], mediated in part by the lypolytic
effects of increased catecholamine and growth hormone secretion [71,72], and diminished concentration of serum insulin
[73,74].

Exercise Versus Diet

Zuti and Golding [67] conducted an especially interesting
study pertaining to differing methods of weight reduction
among middle-aged women. Three experimental groups of 11
women (age range = 25–45 years) each were formed. Treatments were designed to achieve a caloric deficit of 500 kcal per
day over normal activities, as follows: Diet Group, 500 kcal
reduction in dietary intake, no change in regular exercise;
Exercise Group, exercise requiring 500 kcal, no change in caloric
intake; and, Exercise–Diet Group, 250 kcal reduction in diet
and 250 kcal expenditure through exercise. The exercise

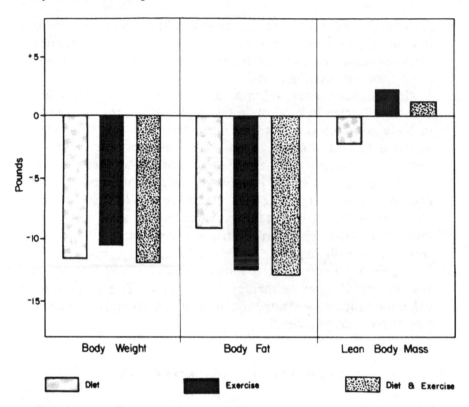

Figure 13. Change in body weight, body fat, and lean body mass following three different methods of weight reduction: diet alone, exercise alone, or combined diet and exercise. Both exercise groups showed significantly greater reductions in body fat than did the diet group, while the diet group demonstrated an undesirable loss in lean body mass. Adapted from Zuti and Golding [67].

program included walking–jogging, bench stepping, and calisthenics. Average changes in body composition, assessed by hydrostatic weighing, are shown in Figure 13. Although all three groups lost weight, the differences among groups were not significant. However, both exercise groups showed significantly greater reductions in body fat than did the Diet Group, while the Diet Group demonstrated an undesirable loss in lean body mass. These data indicate that weight reduction regimens that employ exercise or exercise and caloric restriction produce more desirable changes in body composition than methods using caloric restriction alone.

In summary, exercise with or without caloric restriction appears effective in promoting favorable short-term alterations in body composition. Until recently, however, few data were available to test whether or not these resulting alterations in body composition were "permanent." A follow-up investigation of our earlier studies [59] revealed the disappointing finding that the majority of middle-aged women regress to their preconditioning body weight and fatness when left to exercise on their own [75]. Although caloric restriction has been criticized as a treatment for obesity (i.e., "as few as 5% and probably no more than 20% of all cases achieve long-term success" [76]), perhaps the success of exercise therapy is no better. This emphasizes the importance of sustained motivation and compliance in any weight reducing regimen.*

EXERCISE RECOMMENDATIONS

The effectiveness of exercise training for weight reduction is dependent on sustained compliance and the interplay of several variables including the intensity, frequency, duration, and type of exercise employed (see Chapter 5). In addition, recent studies suggest that environmental factors (i.e., cold exposure) may serve to augment the effect of exercise training on body fat losses.

Research indicates that exercise training of moderate-intensity (e.g., 60–70% of maximal heart rate) and long duration (at least 20 minutes) is optimal for weight loss [77]. During mild-to-moderate intensity aerobic exercise, blood lactate remains low, allowing the individual to continue

*See B. A. Franklin, Exercise program compliance: improvement strategies. In *Behavioral Management of Obesity*, edited by J. Storlie and H. A. Jordan (New York: Spectrum Publications, 1984).

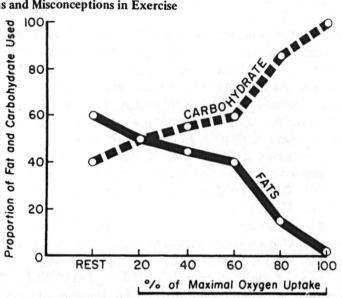

Figure 14. Relative contribution of fat and carbohydrate as a function of exercise intensity, expressed as a percentage of the maximal oxygen uptake (VO_2 max). During mild-to-moderate intensity exercise (e.g., below 60% VO_2 max), fat serves as an important energy substrate. Adapted from Astrand and Rodahl [56].

exercising for a prolonged period of time [78]. In contrast, during high intensity aerobic or anaerobic exercise, lactic acid accumulates rapidly, and fatigue results. Thus, total energy expenditure is maximized with prolonged mild-to-moderate intensity aerobic exercise.

Another reason for recommending mild-to-moderate intensity exercise for weight reduction is the increased utilization of free fatty acids as a fuel source [79]. Although the energy for short periods of high intensity exercise is derived almost entirely from stored carbohydrates (glycogens) in the liver and muscles, mild-to-moderate intensity activities of longer duration use both carbohydrate and fat (Figure 14) [56]. These data highlight the importance of the "long slow distance" concept when targeting body fat as the energy substrate during exercise.

Recent studies in animals [80] and man [81] indicate that caffeine ingestion increases the rate of lipolysis during exercise, as demonstrated by both blood and respiratory exchange data. Similar effects have also been obtained with beta-blockade [82]. These intriguing findings suggest the possibility of favorably increasing fat utilization during exercise training, augmenting body fat losses.

An American College of Sports Medicine position statement [83] suggests that the "minimal threshold" of exercise training for weight and fat reduction includes continuous exercise of at least 20 to 30 minutes duration, an exercise intensity sufficient to expend 300 or more kcal per session, with an exercise frequency of at least three days per week. Exercise programs performed twice a week, regardless of the intensity, duration, or both, appear to be ineffective in reducing body weight and fat stores [84]. In addition, Bjorntorp [2] suggested that exercise training programs under 3 months in duration generally result in minimal or no change in body composition.

The preferred forms of exercise for weight reduction employ large muscle groups, are maintained continuously, and are rhythmical and aerobic in nature, e.g., jogging, running, bicycling, skiing, and swimming. Reduction of body weight and fat stores may even result from brisk walking programs [85], provided the walking duration exceeds 30 minutes [86]. When exercise frequency, intensity, and duration are equated, there appears to be no difference among walking, running, or bicycling as exercise modes to reduce body weight and fat stores [87]. Recreational sports involving sustained total body movement are also effective in promoting a negative energy balance. Table 4 provides the caloric expenditure associated with a variety of recreational activities [88]. In addition, patients should be encouraged to increase physical activity in daily living (Table 5).

Although anaerobic activities do not appear as effective as aerobic exercise in weight reduction programs [79], select anaerobic activities (e.g., weight lifting, sit-ups, etc.) may effect increases in lean body mass. Since lean body mass is related to the metabolic rate, it is apparent that this type of exercise may contribute to energy expenditure. [7]. Anaerobic activities

Table 4. Approximate Metabolic Cost of Common Recreational Activities

Activity	kcal/minute[a]	kcal/hour[a]
Walking (1 mile/hr.)	2.0-2.5	120-150
Walking (2 miles/hr, bicycling (5 miles/hr), billiards, bowling, golf (power cart)	2.5-4.0	150-240
Walking (3 miles/hr), bicycling (6 miles/hr), volleyball, golf (pulling bag cart), archery, badminton (social doubles)	4.0-5.0	240-300
Walking (3.5 miles/hr), bicycling (8 miles/hr), table tennis, golf (carrying clubs), badminton (singles), tennis (doubles), many calisthenics	5.0-6.0	300-360
Walking (4 miles/hr), bicycling (10 miles/hr), ice skating, roller skating	6.0-7.0	360-420
Walking (5 miles/hr), bicycling (11 miles/hr), badminton (competitive), tennis (singles), square dancing, light downhill skiing, water skiing	7.0-8.0	420-480
Jogging (5 miles/hr), bicycling (12 miles/hr), vigorous downhill skiing, basketball, ice hockey, touch football, paddleball	8.0-10.0	480-600
Running (5.5 miles/hr), bicycling (13 miles/hr), squash racquets, handball (social), fencing, basketball (vigorous)	10.0-11.0	600-660
Running (6.0 miles/hr), handball (competitive), squash (competitive)	11.0 plus	660 plus

Adapted from Fox and co-workers [88].
[a]Represents gross caloric expenditure (i.e., includes the resting metabolic needs). Caloric requirements have been calculated for a 70 kg person and must be adjusted proportionately for lighter or heavier weights.

may also promote muscle tone, thereby reducing girth measures.

Finally, recent studies suggest that environmental conditions may influence the effect of exercise on body fat losses. Previous studies have suggested that combined cold exposure and exercise may have synergistic effects on body fat loss [89-93]. Conflicting data, however, were recently reported [94].

Table 5.   Practical Suggestions to Increase Physical Activity in Everyday Living

1. Avoid elevators and escalators—use the steps when possible.

2. Park the car away from the store when shopping.

3. Eliminate home extension phones. (It is estimated that for every extension phone in your home you will save as much as 70 miles of walking a year).

4. Include a 5-minute walk for each television program watched throughout the day.

5. Walk to and from work when possible.

6. Walk when you play golf—avoid motorized carts.

7. Walk the dog more often.

8. Develop and promote "theme" days at home (e.g., no-car day).

9. Use manual instead of power tools and appliances.

10. Store frequently used objects on a different floor of the home.

11. Employ foot and cycle transportation for short neighborhood trips.

Several explanations have been proposed as rationale for the augmented weight loss associated with exercise in the cold. These include loss of body heat, increased metabolism through shivering, increased muscle tension or voluntary body movement, the partial breakdown of fat to ketone bodies, and appetite suppression [89–93]. Since cold exposure is inherent in normal winter recreation, this method of fat loss may prove helpful in treating moderate obesity.

Special Exercise Considerations for the Obese

There are no clear-cut abnormalities in moderate obesity that preclude participation in regular exercise [95]. It is recommended that obese persons, like their normal counterparts, undergo medical screening and exercise tolerance testing prior to beginning an exercise program [37,96–98]. A low incidence of abnormal exercise test responses among the obese suggests that exercise training is relatively safe from a cardiovascular standpoint [97]. Furthermore, our experience with lean and obese middle-aged women suggests that when a relative intensity exercise prescription is employed, the obese individual is no more susceptible to exercise-induced orthopedic injury than is the individual of normal fatness [59].

In contrast to the moderately obese individual, exercise programs for the extremely obese patient, although generally beneficial, can be fraught with certain problems [99,100]. These individuals often have abnormal psychological profiles [99] (e.g., hostility, schizophrenic, paranoid, and manic-depressive tendencies) along with numerous physical limitations including heat intolerance, hyperpnea, low back pain, local musculoskeletal weakness, and incoordination [99–101]. Many patients experience dizziness secondary to hypotension caused by pronounced weight loss [99]. Exercise boredom and poor compliance are also significant problems among the extremely obese. Practical suggestions to cope with these problems and successful training protocols for this patient population are described elsewhere [101,102]. Foss and co-workers [103] reported marked improvement in exercise tolerance among extremely obese patients following a physical conditioning program.

CONCLUSION

The value of physical activity in weight reduction programs has generally been minimized, particularly when compared with dietary intervention. However, exercise with or without caloric restriction offers three important advantages over caloric restriction alone [38]. First, exercise improves musculoskeletal and cardiorespiratory fitness. Second, exercise and recreation can serve as enjoyable leisure-time activities, whereas dieting may be difficult and unpleasant. Third, weight loss through exercise consists primarily of fat as opposed to the loss of water or vital lean tissue which can occur with crash or fad dieting [104].

Unfortunately, man's attempts to regulate his body fatness and proportion through diet and/or exercise have been largely in vain, with poor compliance a big part of the problem [75, 76]. This experience lends additional support to the opinion of an earlier observer who stated, "There is a divinity that shapes our ends" [105].

ACKNOWLEDGEMENT

Special thanks are due to Sheri Waldman for her assistance in the preparation and typing of this manuscript.

REFERENCES

1. Wing, R. R., and Jeffrey, R. J. Outpatient treatments of obesity: A comparison of methodology and results. *Intl. J. Obesity 3*:261-279, 1979.
2. Bjorntrop, P. Physical training in the treatment of obesity. *Intl. J. Obesity 2*:149-156, 1978.
3. Garrow, J. S. *Energy Balance and Obesity in Man* (2nd ed.). Amsterdam, Elsevier, 1978.
4. Mayer, J. *Overweight Causes, Cost, and Control*. Englewood Cliffs, N.J., Prentice-Hall Inc., 1968.
5. Mayer, J., and Bullen, B. A. Nutrition, weight control, and exercise. In *Science and Medicine of Exercise and Sport*. Edited by W. R. Johnson and E. R. Buskirk, New York, Harper and Row, 1974.
6. Garrow, J. S. The regulation of energy expenditure in man. In *Recent Advances in Obesity Research* (Vol. 2). Edited by G. A. Bray, London, Newman, 1978.
7. Thompson, J. K., Jarvie, G. J., Lahey, B. B., et al. Exercise and obesity: Etiology, physiology, and intervention. *Psychological Bulletin 91*:55-79, 1982.
8. Hill, A. V., Long, C. N. H., and Lupton, H. Muscular exercise, lactic acid and the supply and utilization of oxygen. V. The recovery process after exercise in man. *Proc. R. Soc. [B]. 97*:96-138, 1925.
9. Margaria, R., Edwards, H. T., and Dill, D. B. The possible mechanisms of contracting and paying the oxygen debt and the role of lactic acid in muscular contraction. *Am. J. Physiol. 106*:689-715, 1933.

10. Newsholme, E. A. A possible metabolic basis for the control of body weight. *N. Engl. J. Med. 302*:400-405, 1980.
11. Edwards, H. T., Throndike, A., and Dill, D. B. The energy requirement in strenuous exercise. *N. Engl. J. Med. 213*:532-535, 1935.
12. Allen, D. W., and Quigley, B. M. The role of physical activity in the control of obesity. *Med. J. Australia 2*:434-438, 1977.
13. Passmore, R., and Johnson, R. E. Some metabolic changes following prolonged moderate exercise. *Metabolism 9*:452-456, 1960.
14. de Vries, H. A., and Gray, D. E. Aftereffects of exercise upon resting metabolic rate. *Res. Q. 34*:314-321, 1963.
15. Mayer, J., Marshall, N. B., Vitale, J. J., et al. Exercise, food intake and body weight in normal rats and genetically obese adult mice. *Am. J. Physiol. 177*:544-548, 1954.
16. Mayer, J., Roy, P., and Mitra, K. P. Relation between caloric intake, body weight, and physical work: studies in an industrial male population in West Bengal. *Am. J. Clin. Nutr. 4*:169-175, 1956.
17. Dempsey, J. A. Anthropometrical observations on obese and non-obese young men undergoing a program of vigorous physical exercise. *Res. Q. 35*:275-287, 1964.
18. Skinner, J. S., Holloszy, J. O., and Cureton, T. K. Effects of a program of endurance exercises on physical work capacity and anthropometric measuresments of 15-middle-aged men. *Am. J. Cardiol. 14*: 747-752, 1964.
19. Jankowski, L. W., and Foss, M. L. The energy intake of sedentary men after moderate exercise. *Med Sci. Sports 4*:11-13, 1972.
20. Woo, R., Garrow, J. S., and Pi-Sunyer, F. X. Effect of exercise on spontaneous calorie intake in obesity. *Am. J. Clin. Nutr. 36*:470-477, 1982.
21. Woo, R., Garrow, J. S., and Pi-Sunyer, F. X. Voluntary food intake during prolonged exercise in obese women. *Am. J. Clin. Nutr. 36*: 478-484, 1982.
22. Oscai, L. B., and Holloszy, J. O. Effects of weight changes produced by exercise, food restriction, or overeating on body composition. *J. Clin. Invest. 48*:2124-2128, 1969.
23. Stevenson, J. A. F., Box, B. M., Feleki, V., et al. Bouts of exercise and food intake in the rat. *J. Appl. Physiol. 21*:118-122, 1966.
24. Crews, E. L., Fuge, K. W., Oscai, L. B., et al. Weight, food intake, and body composition: Effects of exercise and of protein deficiency. *Am. J. Physiol. 216*:359-363, 1969.
25. Oscai, L. B. The role of exercise in weight control. In *Exercise and Sport Sciences Reviews.* (Vol. 1). Edited by J. H. Wilmore, New York, Academic Press, 1973.

26. Katch, V. L., Martin, R., and Martin, J. Effects of exercise intensity on food consumption in the male rat. *Am. J. Clin. Nutr. 32*:1401-1407, 1979.

27. Baile, C. A., Zinn, M. W., and Mayer, J. Effects of lactate and other metabolites on food intake of monkeys. *Am. J. Physiol. 219*:1606-1613, 1970.

28. Brobeck, J. R. Food intake as a mechanism of temperature regulation. *Yale J. Biol. Med. 20*:545-552, 1948.

29. Belbeck, L. W., and Critz, J. B. Effect of exercise on the plasma concentration of anorexigenic substance in man. *Proc. Soc. Exp. Biol. Med. 142*:19-21, 1973.

30. Kuntzleman, C. *The Exerciser's Handbook.* New York, David McKay Inc., 1978.

31. Mahadeva, K., Passmore, R., and Woolf, B. Individual variations in the metabolic cost of standardized exercise: The effects of food, age, sex and race. *J. Physiol. 121*:225-231, 1953.

32. Dill, D. B. Oxygen used in horizontal and grade walking and running on the treadmill. *J. Appl. Physiol. 20*:19-22, 1965.

33. Margaria, R., Cerretelli, P., Aghemo, P., et al. Energy cost of running. *J. Appl. Physiol. 18*:367-370, 1963.

34. Pugh, L. G. C. E. Oxygen intake in track and treadmill running with observation on the effect of air resistance. *J. Physiol. 207*:823-835, 1970.

35. Howley, E. T., and Glover, M. E. The caloric costs of running and walking one mile for men and women. *Med. Sci. Sports 6*:235-237, 1974.

36. Fellingham, G. W., Roundy, E. S., Fisher, A. G., et al. Caloric cost of walking and running. *Med. Sci. Sports 10*:132-136, 1978.

37. *Guidelines for Graded Exercise Testing and Exercise Prescription.* American College of Sports Medicine. Philadelphia, Lea and Febiger, 1980.

38. Franklin, B. A., and Rubenfire, M. Losing weight through exercise. *J.A.M.A. 244*:377-379, 1980.

39. Hellerstein, H. K., Hirsch, E. Z., Ader, R., et al. Principles of exercise prescription for normals and cardiac subjects. In *Exercise Testing and Exercise Training in Coronary Heart Disease.* Edited by J. P. Naughton and H. K. Hellerstein, New York, Academic Press, 1973.

40. Hernlund, V., and Steinhaus, A. H. Do mechanical vibrators take off or redistribute fat? *J. Assoc. Phys. Ment. Rehabil. 11*:96, 1957.

41. *The Healthy Life: Better Living Through Diet and Exercise.* Edited by N. P. Ross. New York, Time Life Books, 1966.

42. Hellerstein, H. K., and Franklin, B. A. Exercise testing and prescription. In *Rehabilitation of the Coronary Patient*. Edited by N. K. Wenger and H. K. Hellerstein, New York, John Wiley, 1978.

43. Wilmore, J. H., Atwater, A. E., and Maxwell, B. D. Alterations in breast size, shape, and volume with the 21-day Mark Eden "Mark II" bust developer program (abstract) *Med. Sci. Sports 15*:139, 1983.

44. Dunn, K. Exercising at home: Hard work is good work. *Phys. Sportsmed. 9*:110–114, 1981.

45. White, J. R. Changes following ten weeks of exercise using a mini-trampoline in overweight women (abstract). *Med Sci. Sports 12*: 103, 1980.

46. Katch, V. L., Villanacci, J. F., and Sady, S. P. Energy cost of rebound-running. *Res. Q. 52*:269–272, 1981.

47. Getchell, B. *Being Fit: A Personal Guide*. New York, John Wiley and Sons, Inc., 1982.

48. Getchell, B., and Cleary, P. The caloric costs of rope skipping and running. *Phys. Sportsmed. 8*:56–60, 1980.

49. Noland, M., and Kearney, J. T. Anthropometric and densitometric responses of women to specific and general exercise. *Res. Q. 49*:322–328, 1978.

50. Olson, A. L., and Edelstein, E. Spot reduction of subcutaneous adipose tissue. *Res. Q. 39*:647–652, 1968.

51. Carns, M., Schade, M., Liba, M., et al. Segmental volume reduction by localized versus generalized exercise. *Hum. Biol. 32*:370–376, 1960.

52. Roby, F. B. Effects of exercise on regional subcutaneous fat accumulations. *Res. Q. 33*:273–278, 1962.

53. Schade, M., Hellebrandt, F. A., Waterland, J. C., et al. Spot reducing in overweight college women. *Res. Q. 33*:461–471, 1962.

54. Gwinup, G., Chelvam, R., and Steinberg, T. Thickness of subcutaneous fat and activity of underlying muscles. *Ann. Intern. Med. 74*: 408–411, 1971.

55. Katch, F. I., Clarkson, P. M., McBride, T., et al. Preferential effects of abdominal exercise training on regional adipose cell size (abstract). *Med. Sci. Sports 12*:96, 1980.

56. Astrand, P. O., and Rodahl, K. *Textbook of Work Physiology*. New York, McGraw-Hill Book Company, 1970.

57. Zohman, L. R., Kattus, A. A. amd Softmess, D. G. *The Cardiologist's Guide to Fitness and Health Through Exercise*. New York, Simon and Schuster, 1979.

58. Wilmore, J. H. Body composition in sport and exercise: directions for future research. *Med. Sci. Sports 15*:21–31, 1983.

59. Franklin, B., Buskirk, E., Hodgson, J., et al. Effects of physical conditioning on cardiorespiratory function, body composition and serum lipids in relatively normal-weight and obese middle-aged women. *Intl. J. Obesity 3*:97–109, 1979.
60. Akers, R., and Buskirk, E. R. An underwater weighing system utilizing "force cube" transducers. *J. Appl. Physiol. 26*:649–652, 1969.
61. Brozek, J., Grande, F., Anderson, J. T., et al. Densitometric analysis of body composition: revision of some quantitative assumptions. *Ann. N.Y. Acad. Sci. 110*:113–140, 1963.
62. Pollock, M. L., Cureton, T. K., and Greninger, L. Effects of frequency of training on working capacity, cardiovascular function, and body composition of adult men. *Med. Sci. Sports 1*:70–74, 1969.
63. Ribisl, P. M. Effects of training upon the maximal oxygen uptake of middle-aged men. *Int. Zeit. Agnew. Physiol. 27*:154–160, 1969.
64. Wilmore, J. H., Royce, J., Girandola, R. N., et al. Body composition changes with a 10-week program of jogging. *Med. Sci. Sports 2*:113–117, 1970.
65. Bioleau, R. A., Buskirk, E. R., Horstman, D. H., et al. Body composition changes in obese and lean men during physical conditioning. *Med. Sci. Sports 3*:183–189, 1971.
66. Moody, D. L., Wilmore, J. H., Girandola, R. N., et al. The effects of a jogging program on the body composition of normal and obese high school girls. *Med. Sci. Sports 4*:210–213, 1972.
67. Zuti, W. B., and Golding, L. A. Comparing diet and exercise as weight reduction tools. *Phys. Sportsmed. 4*:49–53, 1976.
68. Entenman, C., Goldwater, W. H., Ayres, N. S., et al. Analysis of adipose tissue in relation to body weight loss in man. *J. Appl. Physiol. 13*:129–134, 1958.
69. Young, C. M., and Digiacomo, M. M. Protein utilization and changes in body composition during weight reduction. *Metabolism 14*:1084–1094, 1965.
70. Rodahl, K., Miller, H. I., and Issekutz, B., Jr. Plasma-free fatty acids in exercise. *J. Appl. Physiol. 19*:489–492, 1964.
71. Havel, R. J. Influence of intensity and duration of exercise on supply and use of fuels. In *Muscle Metabolism during Exercise.* Edited by B. Pernow and B. Saltin, New York, Plenum Press, 1971.
72. Glick, S. M., Roth, J., Yalow, R. S., et al. The regulation of growth hormone secretion. *Rec. Progr. Hormone Res. 21*:241–283, 1965.
73. Cochran, B., Marbach, E. P., Poucher, R., et al. Effect of acute muscular exercise on serum immunoreactive insulin. *Diabetes 15*:838–841, 1966.

74. Hunter, W. M., and Sukkar, M. Y. Changes in plasma insulin levels during muscular exercise. *J. Physiol. 196*:110-112, 1968.

75. MacKeen, P. C., Franklin, B. A., Nicholas, W. C., et al. Body composition, physical work capacity and physical activity habits at 18-month follow-up of middle-aged women participating in an exercise intervention program. *Intl. J. Obesity 7*:61-71, 1983.

76. Losing weight It's hard to be good. Medical News. *J.A.M.A. 239*: 1729-1730, 1978.

77. Sharkey, B. J. *Physiological Fitness and Weight Control.* Missoula, Montana, Mountain Press, 1975.

78. Katch, F. I., and McArdle, W. D. *Nutrition, Weight Control, and Exercise.* Boston, Houghton Mifflin, 1977.

79. Girandola, R. N. Body composition changes in women: Effects of high and low exercise intensity. *Arch. Phys. Med. Rehabil. 57*:297-300, 1976.

80. Wilcox, A. R. The effects of caffeine and exercise on body weight, fat-pad weight, and fat-cell size. *Med. Sci. Sports 14*:317-321, 1982.

81. Costil, D. L., Dalsky, G. P., and Fink, W. J. Effects of caffeine ingestion on metabolism and exercise performance. *Med. Sci. Sports 10*: 155-158, 1978.

82. Hossack, K. F., Bruce, R. A., and Kusumi, F. Altered exercise ventilatory responses by apparent propranolol-diminished glucose metabolism: Implications concerning impaired physical training benefit in coronary patients. *Am Heart J. 102*:378-382, 1981.

83. The recommended quantity and quality of exercise for developing and maintaining fitness in healthy adults. American College of Sports Medicine Position Statement. *Med. Sci. Sports 10*:7-9, 1979.

84. Pollock, M. L., Wilmore, J., and Fox, S. M. *Health and Fitness Through Physical Activity.* New York, John Wiley and Sons Inc., 1978.

85. Pollock, M. L., Miller, H. S., Janeway, R., et al. Effects of walking on body composition and cardiovascular function of middle-aged men. *J. Appl. Physiol. 30*:126-130, 1971.

86. Gwinup, G. Effect of exercise alone on the weight of obese women. *Arch. Intern. Med. 135*:676-680, 1975.

87. Pollock, M. L., Dimmick, J., Miller, H. S., et al. Effect of mode of training on cardiovascular function and body composition of adult men. *Med. Sci. Sports 7*:139-145, 1975.

88. Fox, S. M., Naughton, J. P., and Gorman, P. A. Physical activity and cardiovascular health. III. The exercise prescription: frequency and type of activity. *Mod. Concepts Cardiovasc. Dis. 41*:25-30, 1972.

89. O'Hara, W. J., Allen, C., and Shephard, R. J. Loss of body fat during an arctic winter expedition. *Can. J. Physiol. Pharmacol. 55*:1235–1241, 1977.

90. O'Hara, W. J., Allen, C., and Shephard, R. J. Loss of body weight and fat during exercise in a cold chamber. *Eur. J. Appl. Physiol. 37*:205–218, 1977.

91. O'Hara, W. J., Allen, C., and Shephard, R. J. Treatment of obesity by exercise in the cold. *Canad. Med. Ass. J. 117*:773–786, 1977.

92. O'Hara, W. J., Allen, C., Shephard, R. J., et al. Fat loss in the cold—a controlled study. *J. Appl. Physiol. 46*:872–877, 1979.

93. Shephard, R. J., O'Hara, W. J., and Allen, C. Loss of body fat with exercise in the cold. *Medicinea Dello Sport 32*:235–239, 1979.

94. Sheldahl, L. M., Buskirk, E. R., Loomis, J. L., et al. Effects of exercise in cool water on body weight loss. *Intl. J. Obesity 6*:29–42, 1982.

95. Horton, E. S. Diet, muscle metabolism, and capacity for exercise in obesity. In *Recent Advances in Obesity Research* (Vol. 2). Edited by G. A. Bray, London, Newman, 1978.

96. Bjorntorp, P., Sjostrom, L., and Sullivan, L. The role of physical exercise in the management of obesity. In *The Treatment of Obesity*. Edited by J. F. Munro, Baltimore, Md., University Park Press, 1979.

97. DeVore, P. A., and Nemiro, D. D. Exercise testing of obese subjects. *Phys. Sportsmed. 8*:47–54, 1980.

98. Foss, M. L., Lampman, R. M., Watt, E., et al. Initial work tolerance of extremely obese patients. *Arch. Phys. Med. Rehabil. 56*:63–67, 1975.

99. Goodman, C., and Kenrick, M. Physical fitness in relation to obesity. *Obesity and Bariatric Medicine 4*:12–15, 1975.

100. Kenrick, M. M., Ball, M. F., and Canary, J. J. Exercise and weight reduction in obesity. *March. Phys. Med. Rehabil. 53*:323–327, 340, 1972.

101. Foss, M. L. Exercise prescription and training programs for obese subjects. In *Proceedings of the Third International Congress on Obesity*. London, Newman Publishing Co., 1981.

102. Foss, M. L., Lampman, R. M., and Schteingart, D. Physical training program for rehabilitating extremely obese patients. *Arch. Phys. Med. Rehabil. 57*:425–429, 1976.

103. Foss, M. L., Lampman, R. M., and Schteingart, D. E. Extremely obese patients: Improvements in exercise tolerance with physical training and weight loss. *Arch. Phys. Med. Rehabil. 61*:119–124, 1980.

104. Fineberg, S. K. The realities of obesity and fad diets. *Nutrition Today 7*:23–26, 1972.

105. Shakespeare, W. *Hamlet, Prince of Denmark*, Act V, Sc. 2.

5

Exercise Testing and Training for the Obese

Merle L. Foss and Deborah A. Strehle

INTRODUCTION

Exercise has "come of age." It is now researched and advocated by many health professionals and citizens as a valuable tool in the ongoing fight against pandemic obesity [1-9].

Exercise has been recognized for centuries as an outlet for ingested energy to maintain an ideal percentage of body fat. Figure 1 illustrates that energy can only enter the metabolic system through eating and/or drinking, i.e., food energy (E food). Fat stores accumulate when food intake exceeds the combined energy conversions to heat and motion (physical activity). The stored fat will be utilized during periods of extended activity when energy needs exceed food intake. In

$E_{(food)} = E_{(heat)} + E_{(move)} \pm E_{(fat)}$

- Positive caloric "balance"

$E_{(food)} > \Sigma E_{(heat)} + E_{(move)}$ So $+ E_{(fat)}$

- Negative caloric "balance"

$E_{(food)} < \Sigma E_{(heat)} + E_{(move)}$ So $- E_{(fat)}$

- Isocaloric ("true") balance

$E_{(food)} = E_{(heat)} + E_{(move)}$ So $E_{(fat)}$ **SAME**

- Negative "balance" over time   So $- E_{(fat)}$ **LOSS**

- Best achieved by combining

$\downarrow E_{(food)}$ through calorie restricted **DIET**

$\uparrow E_{(move)}$ through daily activities and **EXERCISE**

Figure 1. Basic energy balance equations.

theory, an obese person should lose fat tissue during inadequate food intake (negative caloric balance) and will gain fat tissue during excessive food intake (positive caloric balance).

Energy requirements can vary in individuals depending upon amount of activity within their lifestyles. Furthermore, energy balance may be manipulated with exercise alone or in combination with dietary intake to decrease, stabilize, or even increase body fat stores [10,11]. The interaction of these variables is the basis for most weight loss program recommendations. A major source of energy expenditure should be in the form of daily activities combined with consistent, progressive exercise [12]. In addition, a combination of reduced food energy intake and increased energy output will cause a reduction in body fat stores when applied over time [13]. The consequences and limitations of obesity are recognized [14] and appropriate precautions must be taken (see Chapter 6, "Exercise Concerns and Precautions for the Obese"). The need for widespread acceptance of therapeutic exercise in obesity is evident. Allied health care professionals have previously limited their role in prescribing exercise programs to obese clients for various reasons. One problem has simply been lack of confidence related to the malpractice and litigative risks associated with exercise testing and training the obese. In addition, the public has been misled due to many existing myths and misconceptions related to exercise. Chapter 4 "Exercise Intervention for Weight Control: Myths and Misconceptions," addresses this problem.

Despite these inhibiting factors in exercising the obese, many proponents of therapeutic exercise strongly believe that consistent participation is the only way to effectively reduce and maintain ideal body weight. In examining the following benefits of exercise, it is clearly a valuable therapeutic adjunct.

Physiological Benefits
1. increased aerobic capacity
2. decreased resting heart rate
3. decreased blood pressure
4. reduced serum cholesterol and triglycerides
5. increased muscle strength and endurance
6. improved sleep

Psychosocial Benefits
1. reduced tension, anxiety, and fatigue
2. enhanced feelings of well-being and euphoria
3. improved self-image
4. opportunities for shared activity with family and friends
5. motivation and incentive to participate in group exercise and community events

The process outlined in Table 1 summarizes how exercise contributes to weight loss. These recommendations apply to all categories of obesity, ranging from apparently healthy individuals to those people considered high risk for developing coronary heart disease. This chapter examines risks involved in exercise testing the obese and addresses specific ways to prescribe a personal, safe, and effective weight loss and maintenance program. In addition, practical procedures are presented in

Table 1. How Exercise Contributes to Weight Loss

1. Exercise is a valid, safe and effective adjunct therapy for the obese

2. Major contributions of exercise:
   Improvement of physical fitness
   Enhancement of psychological fitness and self-esteem
   Promotion of fat weight reduction

3. Major reasons exercise is not practiced by obese:
   Prevailing myths and misconceptions
   Fear due to poor understanding
   Lack of confidence to prescribe or recommend
   Concern about malpractice or liability litigation

4. Ways to overcome these inhibiting factors:
   Counter myths and misconceptions with documented facts
   Educate obese patients and clients
   Teach procedures for developing exercise programs
   Describe risk management strategies

order to alleviate some of the limitations associated with exercise testing and training the obese, such as anxiety and litigative risks. The following points are discussed: (1) exercise risk appraisal, (2) exercise testing, (3) exercise prescription, and (4) training principles for the obese.

EXERCISE RISK APPRAISAL

One of the first strategies in managing risks associated with exercising the obese is knowing the client. Three major categories are examined in this section: weight classification, age classification, health status and cardiovascular risk appraisal. In addition, general guidelines for managing the obese with known heart disease are presented.

Weight Classification

Assessing the degree of obesity will guide health care professionals through the first steps of choosing effective techniques for exercise testing and prescription. Three major categories may be considered:

slightly obese	120	percent of ideal body weight
moderately obese	130	percent of ideal body weight
extremely obese	150	percent of ideal body weight

Ideal body weight refers to the most recent tables published by the Metropolitan Life Insurance Company [15]. Although this method is arbitrary, it has the advantage of popularity, ease of interpretation, and comparability to other obesity studies that have incorporated these standards.

In classifying the degree of obesity for purposes of exercise testing, this system suffices although it is not necessarily the specific weight category that will direct the strategy of exercise therapy. In fact, it is possible that someone classified as moderate may be at a higher coronary risk than someone classified as extremely obese. Therefore, a reasonable and prudent approach is to develop strategies with consideration of the inherent risks and, at the same time, maintain adaptability in delivering services to meet individual needs.

The slightly obese individual should be managed according to the guidelines established by the American College of Sports Medicine [16] for exercise testing and training apparently healthy adults, with respect to factors such as age and coronary risk status. Individuals classified as moderately or extremely obese, however, have increased coronary risk, as well as a greater chance of musculoskeletal complications. Therefore, as the degree of obesity increases, additional concerns arise, not only in terms of health risks, but in the administration of exercise tests. Electrode placement, poor balance of the subject, and artifact on the electrocardiogram make exercise testing more difficult. Some of these practical problems are discussed in the section of this chapter on Exercise Testing.

Age Classification

The American College of Sports Medicine has established specific guidelines for age classification in graded exercise testing [16]. Coronary risk factors, and thus risks in exercise testing, increase with age. On the other hand, earlier evidence indicates that ischemic changes in persons under age 35, without other coronary risk factors are less than one case per hundred [17]. For this reason, the American College of Sports Medicine has used age 35 to differentiate age classifications. According to established standards of practice in the health care field, the methods and precautions for exercise testing and training adults in these two age groups are clearly and specifically outlined. Assessment and management of exercise programs for obese children involve additional considerations, which are not included in the scope of this chapter.

Health Status and Cardiovascular Risk Appraisal

Next, the individual's current health status should be evaluated. A physician must assess general health and establish the client as apparently healthy, healthy with elevated cardiovascular risks (i.e., asymptomatic in regards to heart disease), or diagnosed heart disease. Table 2 presents a schema to determine the approach to stress testing with consideration to degree of obesity, age, and health/cardiovascular status. This approach emphasizes the importance of managing each client individually and recognizing the combined effect of specific risk factors.

Primary cardiovascular risk factors include family history of heart disease, hypertension, hypercholesterolemia, cigarette smoking, elevated serum triglyceride and glucose levels, abnormal resting and /or exercise electrocardiogram. Stress, inactivity, obesity, and diet are also risk factors which are lifestyle in nature [18]. Recommended standards for classifying patients and clients into these groups have been published [17].

Health professionals need to be aware that these recommendations indicate a wide variety of clinical tests for determining coronary risk. The graded exercise stress test is included in this test battery and should be administered to all adults when beginning a routine exercise program.

According to Cooper, it is important to evaluate an individual's level of physical fitness prior to an exercise program for the following reasons [19]:

1. to determine the current level of physical fitness and overall health status,
2. to objectively evaluate individual responses to exercise training,
3. to medically screen for ischemic heart disease,
4. to determine work capacity for designing an exercise prescription.

While epidemiological studies have established that persons having one or more risk factors are statistically predisposed to coronary heart disease, it is not documented that this absolutely places them at a greater risk for exercise testing and training [18]. This poses the question of whether or not the obese person with one or more coronary risk factors actually needs a traditional graded exercise test. Although current research has not established a concrete link between elevated coronary risk factors and the degree of risk with exercise, a cautious approach in exercising the obese must be taken.

Obese persons with known coronary heart disease, but without functional disability (i.e., asymptomatic) present special problems in exercise risk management. An extremely conservative approach must be taken with these individuals, such as a physician-supervised cardiac rehabilitation exercise program. The American Heart Association Committee on Exercise advocates regular, vigorous exercise as an important therapeutic tool in rehabilitating patients suffering from angina pectoris and those recovering from a myocardial infarction or heart surgery [17,18].

Table 2. Suggested Scheme for Managing Risks of Exercise Testing and Training of Obese Patients and Clients

Categories	Age (yrs)	CHD risk factors	Graded stress test, ECG	Supervised initial training
Slightly obese[a]				
Apparently healthy	<35	No major ones[d]	Optional	Optional
	>35	No major ones	Optional	Optional
Elevated risk for developing heart disease	<35	Certain combinations[e]	Recommended	Optional
	>35	Certain combinations	Recommended	Recommended
Known heart disease	<35	With or without	REQUIRED	REQUIRED
	>35	With or without	REQUIRED	REQUIRED
Moderately obese[b]				
Apparently healthy	<35	No major ones	Optional	Optional
	>35	No major ones	Recommended	Optional

Elevated risk for developing heart disease	<35	Certain combinations	Recommended	Recommended
	>35	Certain combinations	REQUIRED	Recommended
Known heart disease	<35	With or without	REQUIRED	REQUIRED
	>35	With or without	REQUIRED	REQUIRED
Extremely obese[c]				
All categories	Any	With or without	REQUIRED	REQUIRED

[a]Defined as 120% to 130% of "ideal" body weight as determined from Metropolitan Life Insurance Company body weight for height standards [15].

[b]Defined as 131% to 150% of "ideal" body weight.

[c]Defined as 151% to 175% of "ideal" body weight.

[d]No hypertension, hypercholesterolemia and/or hypertriglyceridemia, cigarette smoking or resting ECG abnormalities.

[e]Any major risk factor alone or in combination with secondary risk factors, especially hypertension, ECG abnormalities and sedentary living habits.

EXERCISE TESTING

The American Heart Association Committee on Exercise has defined four major objectives for testing apparently healthy adults [17]:

1. to establish a diagnosis of overt or latent heart disease,
2. to evaluate responses to conditioning and/or preventive programs,
3. to evaluate cardiovascular functional capacity, particularly as a means for screening prior to strenuous work or exercise,
4. to increase individual motivation for entering and adhering to exercise programs.

The primary objective for the health care professional in exercise testing the obese is to determine the individual's functional responses and limitations to exercise. This is important data for designing a safe, effective exercise program.

This section examines several exercise testing modalities and discusses the pros and cons of each. Other references fully describe the specific procedures for graded exercise testing [16,17]; however, an important objective for the health care professional is to select a protocol that most accurately and effectively assesses the obese subject.

Selecting the Exercise Test

Obese subjects present certain inherent problems in testing due to their excess weight. One problem is the fact that they are at an increased coronary risk, so precautions must be considered while administering any graded exercise test. In addition, technical difficulties often interfere with the monitoring of cardiovascular function. For example, electrical interference on the electrocardiogram is very common and heart sounds are difficult to hear with the stethoscope due to thick layers of adipose tissue. Balance, coordination, and sometimes profuse sweating also present problems during the exercise test.

The exercise test protocol should be selected with the following considerations:

1. to measure heart rate, blood pressure, and breathing responses to exercise;
2. to monitor signs and symptoms of exertional distress;
3. to document undue anxieties;
4. to allow individuals to regain lost confidence;
5. to teach principles of pulse rate monitoring;
6. to obtain data for exercise prescription and program development.

Remember, exercise testing in this setting is not a diagnostic tool for heart disease. The purpose is to evaluate physiological responses to exercise so that effective conditioning programs can be designed. Further, baseline data is established so improvements are documented over time.

Four exercise test protocols that meet all of the above objectives are: (1) a simple walking test, (2) a step test, (3) two treadmill protocols, and (4) a bicycle ergometer test.

Walking Test. Table 3 outlines a non-traditional walking test that can be used to test slightly obese, apparently healthy adults. A primary disadvantage of this test is that it is not a graded exercise test with an electrocardiogram, therefore continuous monitoring is not possible. Since body weight is carried while walking a slow to moderate pace, this test is practical, yielding valuable insights into individual capabilities and responses to walking. Table 4 provides examples of using heart rates from a variable pace walking test to determine the subject's training speed when prescribing exercise intensity.

The exercise technician monitors the subject through various stages of the walk, making notations of blood pressure, heart rate, and any visible signs of distress. Another responsibility of the technician is to assist the subject in maintaining the proper pace of walking. This test should be conducted on a level grade, i.e., a long hallway, open room, gymnasium, a standard 440 yard track, outdoor parking lot or sidewalk.

Table 3.   Variable Pace Walking Test for Selected
Obese Subjects

Duration (min)	Pace speed			Distance/3 min	
	mph	km/h	min/mile	yards	meters
3	2.0	3.2	30	176	193
3	2.5	4.0	24	220	241
3	3.0	4.8	20	264	289
3	3.5	5.6	17.1	308	337
3	4.0	6.4	15	352	385

Procedure:
1.   Determine standing Resting Heart Rate (RHR), Breathing Rate (BR), and Blood Pressure (BP).
2.   Leave BP cuff on.
3.   Determine Exercise Heart Rate (EHR), BR and BP immediately after each 3 minute walk pace that easily can be performed.
4.   Note signs and symptoms of exertional distress, anxiety statements, and complaints.
5.   Allow 3 minutes of recovery. Check HR, BR, and BP.
6.   Teach subject to self-monitor EHR (10 sec count × 6 = bpm).

Total time required to administer this test is approximately 30 minutes, which includes preliminary instructions, recording of measurements, and recovery time.

Step Test. One of the earliest exercise tests designed was the Harvard Step Test [20]. After stepping up and down on a bench for a specified time, the subject's fitness level is determined by measuring resting and recovery heart rates. One and three minute step tests have been developed, using a standard height for the step box or bench [20]. Since the existing procotols were developed using non-obese subjects, modifications in the height of the step and stepping cadence may be necessary for obese subjects. Particular attention should be given to the strain on legs, knees, and ankles when administering a step test to obese subjects. Although this test is simple and quick, requiring very little special equipment or skill to administer, it does have a few disadvantages. Besides leg strain, there is no continuous electrocardiographic monitoring. For high risk subjects, this is a major consideration.

Table 4. Example of Using Exercise Heart Rates (EHR) from Variable Pace Walking Test to Determine Best Initial Walk Speed

Pace speed (mph)	EHR[a] (beats/min)	ΔHR/CR (percent)	EHR/THR[b] ratio	Rating of pace	Miles/20 min
2.0	90	14	0.65	Too slow	0.66
2.5	102	26	0.74	Slow	0.83
3.0	120	43	0.87	Better	1.00
3.5	138	60[c]	1.00	Best	1.16
4.0	156	77	1.13	Too fast	1.32

[a]Exercise heart rate immediately post exercise by pulse counting for 10 seconds ×6 = beats per minute.
[b]Target heart rate at 60 percent of CR for 40 year old subject; Est. MHR = 220 – age = 220 –40 = 180, RHR = 75, CR = Est. MHR – RHR = 180 –75 = 105, THR = 0.60 (CR) + RHR = 0.60 (105) + 75 = 138.
[c]ΔHR = EHR–RHR = 138 – 75 = 63, ΔHR/CR = 63/105 = .60 × 100 = 60%.

Treadmill Testing. Using a treadmill and electrocardiogram, the most accurate indication of a subject's exercise capabilities can be assessed. With continuous monitoring of heart rate and rhythm, as well as blood pressure, the subject's physiological responses to exertion can be thoroughly evaluated. Since walking is a training mode many obese will select, it is advantageous to use a testing mode that involves walking.

Although treadmill testing with an electrocardiogram has these advantages, some problems are evident. For example, blood pressure is difficult to hear over the treadmill sounds. Many overweight subjects lack coordination and balance while treadmill walking/jogging, feel dizzy and even trip during the test. It is not uncommon for the treadmill conveyor belt to be stopped due to a subject's excess weight.

Another problem encountered in treadmill testing obese subjects is their inability to maintain the workloads of the test at steeper grades due to leg fatigue. Careful selection and adaptation of the test protocol can alleviate this problem, to an extent. During non-weight supported exercise, such as the step test, or treadmill walking, the work rate requirement is a function of body weight times the height the body is raised in a given period of time. When carrying the body on an inclined or vertical plane, obese individuals tend to experience leg fatigue before the cardiovascular system has been taxed. Therefore, a test protocol which increases speed, rather than elevation, will reduce leg strain, allowing the subject to reach higher workloads.

Two popular protocols are the Balke and Bruce tests. The Bruce Protocol [19], designed for healthy adults, begins at a 10% elevation and speed of 1.7 mph. Every three minutes the treadmill is elevated by 2%, as the speed also increases. These rapid increments in workload are intended to reach the test endpoint in a relatively short period of time; however, many obese subjects cannot handle even three minutes of this test. Balance and coordination problems, along with leg strain, are exacerbated.

The Balke Protocol [19] is an example of a treadmill test that can be easily adapted for the obese subject. Beginning at a horizontal grade, the treadmill is elevated by 3% every three minutes, with a constant speed of 3.0 mph throughout the test. The speed may be adjusted to accommodate the walking pace of obese subjects (e.g., 2.5 mph). Another modification would be to reduce the grade increments to 2% every three minutes. These adaptations reduce leg strain and offer the flexibility to meet the wide range of fitness levels encountered in obese populations.

Bicycle Ergometer Test. A bicycle ergometer test is the most accommodating of all the preceeding tests mentioned, because the subject's body weight is supported by the bicycle seat, reducing the impact on tendons, joints, and ligaments. The majority of subjects, however, do not use cycling as their primary activity mode. This reduces some accuracy in evaluating the physiological responses to conditioning, especially for walking and jogging programs.

In selecting a bicycle protocol, the YMCA and Åstrand Bicycle Tests are the most common choices [20]. The YMCA protocol is a submaximal test that is very easy to administer;

however, it has not been designed to include electrocardiographic monitoring. With the addition of an electrocardiogram either of these protocols are adequate testing procedures.

A few concerns should be brought to the attention of the test administrator. The size of the bicycle seat must be large enough to accommodate the posterior of the obese subject. In addition, the bicycle needs to have enough distance between the seat and handlebars so the obese subject can mount the bicycle and comfortably pedal. Movement of the subject's torso while pedaling may create electrical interference on the electrocardiogram, which can be reduced by adjusting the seat and handlebars so that there is minimal extraneous movement.

General Considerations

Although exercise testing is a critical step in designing safe, effective physical conditioning and weight loss programs, it is clearly a complicated process. Obviously, professionals involved in stress testing obese populations must be sensitive and flexible, adapting standard procedures to circumvent problems and meet the individual needs of the obese. The skills of a professional trained in exercise testing are obviously required.

Professionals certified by the American College of Sports Medicine as exercise technologists or exercise specialists have been trained to recognize signs of exertional distress, symptoms that indicate serious complications, and the criteria for terminating a test. Accurate blood pressure measurement, electrocardiogram interpretation, and emergency cardiopulmonary resuscitation are essential skills for test administrators, whether they are health spa personnel, YMCA staff, exercise physiologists, or allied health professionals.

In addition to trained, expert staff, standard emergency procedures for stress testing obese populations must be followed. In establishing and rehearsing these procedures consider the additional complication of managing a large body mass in the event that a subject loses consciousness. Removing the person from the treadmill for defibrillation, carrying the body down or up stairs, or any maneuvering of body mass will be difficult with subjects weighing 250–300 pounds. Anticipation of these problems may save a person's life.

Accurate and safe methods to assess cardiovascular function and overall tolerance to exercise form the foundation of a physical conditioning program for weight control. A variety of traditional procedures may be used, as long as there is consideration of the modifications necessary to accommodate the needs of the obese. Available equipment, facilities, and staff, as well as time limitations and health status of the population served, will determine which procedures and modifications are most practical in a given setting. The primary objective of designing a conditioning program based on individual responses to monitored exercise should be kept in mind as these management decisions are made.

EXERCISE PRESCRIPTION

Individualized exercise prescription designed for a variety of patients and clients is a recent innovation in health care. This section covers essential components of the exercise prescription with respect to the special needs of the obese. Procedures for post-coronary patients [18,21] and apparently healthy, middle-aged adults [17,22] can be applied to designing an exercise prescription for obese subjects [23]. In general, the approach is to (1) assimilate exercise test data to formulate individualized exercise prescriptions, and (2) adjust the exercise prescription for maximal effectiveness.

Developing exercise prescriptions to insure adherence and compliance at the beginning of a program, as well as throughout the maintenance phase, must also be considered [24]. Similar benefits can be achieved with a variety of modalities; therefore the subject is encouraged to choose one or more activities of personal preference. Noncompetitive activities are recommended from the standpoint of safety and prevention of injury [23], since they are usually performed at a low intensity for prolonged periods. Physiologically, the best exercises are ones that involve large muscle groups, are rhythmic in nature, and stimulate adaptations of the cardiovascular system [25].

Exercise Modalities

In selecting the type of exercise to be used for weight loss, it is important to emphasize the role of aerobic activity in burning calories. Just as a fire fuels better when fed oxygen, the body burns stored fat when involved in aerobic exercise. Although a sound exercise program should include activities which enhance all fitness components, individuals desiring to maximize weight loss efforts should spend most of their exercise time in aerobic activities.

A few other considerations are pertinent in selecting a modality: (1) participant's interest, (2) individual limitations, (3) avoiding injury and insuring safety, and (4) potential for long-term adherence.

This section will discuss some of the popular exercise modalities, stressing the specific needs of the obese.

Walking. An excellent recommendation for obese persons is a routine walking program. It has been shown to be an effective exercise mode for both moderate [26–29] and extremely obese [29,30] individuals. In addition, walking has documented benefits for slightly obese [31] and normal weight [32] individuals in decreasing body fat and improving cardiovascular function.

Convenience is a major advantage in that no equipment or facilities are required, except for supportive, well-cushioned shoes. A walking program does not require any special skills or abilities. It is a safe activity because intensity is easily regulated and orthopedic strains are minimal. Walking can also be a fun, social activity if groups meet and select scenic routes. Many parks have walking/jogging trails that wind through beautiful wooded areas. Groups of employees can use lunch hours to walk outside or through hallways, taking the social time to exercise rather than eat. In summary, walking improves cardiorespiratory fitness and is a lifelong activity that lends itself to self management.

Stationary Cycling. Although this modality has slightly less universal appeal than walking because it requires equipment and it tends to become boring, it offers other advantages [33]. As an indoor activity, stationary cycling circumvents the weather elements. Use of alternate muscle groups provides a cross-training effect, so cycling is an excellent adjunct to walking. As a weight-supported activity, orthopedic problems are minimized with this training mode. It is particularly effective for the extremely obese who begin at very low levels of cardiovascular fitness. By reading or watching television while stationary cycling, many individuals find that they enjoy the time spent on the bicycle. In fact, some people will schedule cycling during the evening news or a favorite soap opera as a convenient way to fit exercise into their daily routine.

Swimming and Water Activities. When participants express an interest in aquatic-type activities, swimming, water jogging, or water aerobics/calisthenics should be encouraged. Since fat weight is displaced in the water, the musculoskeletal system is not burdened with the strain of excess body weight. Therefore, orthopedic problems are significantly reduced.

Swimming adds variety to other activities, and again serves as an excellent cross-training method. On the other hand, target heart rates may be difficult to sustain during swimming unless the skill level of the participant is intermediate to advanced. One major obstacle with swimming is simply the need for a year-round swimming pool. Another problem for the obese is finding proper attire that is both functional and modest in the water.

Other aquatic-activities, such as water aerobics, calisthenics, or jogging programs, are excellent alternatives to swimming. These programs are fun, especially when choreographed to music. It is not necessary that participants know how to swim nor even to submerge their heads. Therefore, many individuals who are afraid of water, or simply do not wish to get their hair wet, may find these activities enjoyable.

Jogging. This popular activity may be recommended to those individuals categorized as "slightly obese" [34] who have been on a consistent walking and/or walk-jog program. These participants should be free from lower body orthopedic problems, since injury risks are greater with jogging than for brisk walking. Intensity is difficult to regulate, until proper pacing is learned. Jogging should not be prescribed as an initial activity for moderately and extremely obese subjects. These individuals usually have elevated perceptions of exertion and would be unable to continue the activity for the required duration. As with walking, jogging is a fun way to see various sights and socialize. Be creative with your walking and jogging programs. Create support groups of walking and jogging clubs for those who thrive on the energy of others. In summary, jogging has many of the same advantages as walking; however, it is not considered optimal for all obese clients due to orthopedic strain.

Calisthenics-Stretching. As a supplement to routine aerobic exercise, these activities are recommended for all obese clients to improve total body fitness, i.e., the strength and flexibility components [27,30,25]. No special equipment is required, very little space is needed, and these exercises can be practiced in a wide variety of settings, such as a living room, hotel room, or outdoors. Calisthenics and stretching can be assigned as self-help regimens to be practiced at home each day and/or included as part of supervised, group sessions. Health professionals should emphasize dynamic movements using large body parts such as arms and legs for the warm-up phase. This allows the participant to prepare both physically and psychologically for aerobic activity.

Leading calisthenic and stretching exercises is a good opportunity to teach how various exercises benefit each body part, differentiating between the flexibility and strengthening exercises. Instruction on proper techniques and posture during these exercises is important for avoiding injury. Most obese participants enjoy a routine set to music and prefer a repetitive series of exercises, so they can observe their improvements in coordination and endurance over time. It is important for the exercise leader to be patient with participants, as many of the exercises take more time for them to learn and are difficult to perform because of bulky body parts.

Weight Training. For individuals who wish to realize significant improvements in strength, this activity should be considered as an important adjunct to a regular aerobics program. It is recommended for obese persons with poor strength and/or muscular endurance. Weight training is very effective for rehabilitation from injuries and to build strength for protection of joints, such as the knees, hips, and spine. It can be practiced at home with inexpensive dumbbell and barbell weights or on the more elaborate equipment available at local health clubs. Although cardiovascular fitness and weight loss are not always achieved with weight training alone, other important benefits can be realized. Weight training builds and tones muscles, protecting the body from loss of lean body weight during long periods of dietary restriction or semi-starvation. This will also alleviate some of the sagging skin that results from excessive weight loss. Obese clients need direct, individualized instruction on general weight training principles and proper lifting techniques, especially when using free weights, to insure chances of success and reduce the risks of injury. Weight training has been a popular exercise mode with men; however, increasing numbers of women are now enjoying the benefits of weight training. Since men tend to be attracted to weight training programs, this should be a strong consideration for a target audience that has a large percentage of men.

Rhythmic Movement. This activity includes aerobic dance, jazz dance, modern dance, calisthenics, marching, and any other upbeat-type movement performed to the tempo of music. Aerobic exercise in this form is usually done in groups creating a fun and playful atmosphere, depending on the enthusiasm of the instructor. Cardiovascular benefits may be realized if the frequency, intensity and duration requirements are met. Potential problems with this type of activity include (1) inconsistent leadership quality, (2) strenuous routines causing the subject to exceed their training heart rate, (3) relatively high cost, and (4) clothing requirements that may be unacceptable for obese persons.

Recreational Games. Court games such as squash, bad-
minton, basketball, tennis, volleyball, racquetball, and handball
can be used to improve cardiovascular fitness when played
regularly with adequate intensity and duration. Some games
such as softball, golf and bowling do not qualify as aerobic,
even though they do provide enjoyable social benefits. Recreational activities are not recommended as initial training
modalities because of injury risks and difficulty in regulating
exercise intensity, especially in a competitive situation. Other
problems include age limitations and dependence on equipment
and facilities as well as finding other team members to play the
game. The social interactions, variety, and fun are advantages
which should be considered when planning group activities.
Recreational games can be incorporated into a program to break
up the routine and expose participants to a variety of activities.
Static stretching is important before recreational activities to
improve flexibility and prevent possible injuries from the
sudden intense bursts of activity that often occur in games. If
properly administered and supervised, these activities improve
dynamic strength, coordination, and balance. Further, games
foster a team spirit, promoting group cohesiveness.

Summary. Many options and choices of exercise modes are
available when designing fun, effective training programs for the
obese. The challenge is to meet the needs of the participants,
based on the results of the screening and evaluation process, as
well as personal interests and lifestyle.

Components of Exercise Prescription

Frequency. Exercising three to five times per week is
recommended to develop and maintain fitness [19]. Improvement tends to plateau when exercise frequency exceeds three
days per week; however, the goal of expending calories strongly
indicates the need for greater frequency of training than is
required simply for developing and maintaining fitness. Another
point to recognize is that fitness gains decrease proportionally

as orthopedic risks increase, so too much exercise could be harmful and counterproductive. The therapist must consider the subject's fitness level and willingness to commit time for exercise, and balance these factors with the goal of burning calories.

For example, a reasonable goal would be 20 minutes of walking 3-5 times per week. This goal would burn about 400 calories per week, averaging approximately 50 calories per day. The time required to implement this program is one to one and a half hours per week. At this level of participation, an individual can be safely introduced to regular exercise. Until the person is physically and psychologically prepared for more exercise, restriction of food intake will be critical for producing significant weight loss since it is necessary to burn 3500 calories to lose one pound of fat weight.

Duration. The American College of Sports Medicine recommends 20 minutes of continuous aerobic activity to achieve cardiovascular benefits [17]. Obese persons may experience difficulty performing continuous exercise due to muscle fatigue, anxiety, or elevated perceptions of exertion. A modified version of interval training may be used to give brief periods of recovery by slowing down, rather than discontinuing exercise. Exercise sessions should be at least three minutes, while rest periods should be as short as possible (e.g., 30-60 seconds).

Intensity. This component of an exercise prescription must be carefully formulated based on age, medications and current fitness level. Training heart rate (THR) is used as a guide to monitor exercise intensity during activity.

The Karvonen formula [36] is used to calculate THR:

1. RHR = Resting Heart Rate
2. HRmax = Maximum Heart Rate = 220 – age
3. HRR = HRmax – RHR
4. Recommended percent = 60–90%
5. THR = (Recommended percent × HRR) + RHR

Table 5. Potential Range of Generalized Low Intensity (60% of HRR) THR Assignments Due to Individual Variability about the Mean of Age-Related Maximum Heart Rate Estimates

Age (years)	Est. MHR range[a] mean ($\bar{X}$) ± 10 bpm	THR (low)[b] bpm	THR ($\bar{X}$)[c] bpm	THR (high)[d] bpm
20	190–210	144	150	156
30	180–200	138	144	150
40	170–190	132	138	144
50	160–180	126	132	138
60	150–170	120	126	132
70	140–160	114	120	126

[a] Age-related mean ($\bar{X}$) maximum heart rate (est. MHR) estimated by 220 – age.
[b] Target heart rate using low value of est. MHR and RHR = 75 bpm.
[c] Target heart rate using mean value of est. MHR and RHR = 75 bpm.
[d] Target heart rate using high value of est. MHR and RHR = 75 bpm.

The American College of Sports Medicine recommends exercising between 60–90% of heart rate reserve (HRR) [37], depending on the age and health status of the individual. An intensity of 60% is a low level that is advised for individuals with known heart disease, while 90% is recommended for conditioned athletes. See Table 5 for potential range of generalized low intensity (60%) training heart rate assignments based on age predicted maximum heart rates. For the slightly to moderately obese without known heart disease, an intensity of 70–75% would be an appropriate recommendation.

Summary. In designing an exercise prescription, the frequency, intensity, and duration of exercise sessions are combined to formulate a program that is suitable for the individual. Consideration must be given to the person's time schedule, preferences, orthopedic limitations, cardiovascular health status, fitness level, and weight loss goals.

TRAINING PRINCIPLES FOR THE OBESE

Some major principles that pertain to the organization and delivery of training programs for obese clients follow. These principles reflect both standard training principles and methods that have been adapted through trial and error.

1. Individuals ranging from slightly obese to extremely obese can be effectively and safely trained using modified versions of standard physical training methods.

2. Modifications in training programs should reflect known limitations of the obese as well as other concerns and precautions (Chapter 6 "Exercise Concerns and Precautions for the Obese").

3. Physical training programs should emphasize rehabilitation to higher levels of wellness and quality of life rather than only prepare for recreational athletics. In fact, the competitive aspects should be deemphasized.

4. Individualized training programs and exercise prescriptions should be developed in detail using all available information as provided by the subject. This includes previous medical history, physical exam, and any exercise test results.

5. Obese clients can be trained using a variety of exercise modes. Health professionals should emphasize those modes that adapt best to individuals based on their personal reports.

6. Training modalities and methods taught and practiced by clients should be those which will fit into their personal lifestyle and they may continue after completing the formal, supervised programs.

7. Training programs and exercise prescriptions should be developed around the nucleus of fun and enjoyment. This insures improved adherence, compliance, and long term maintenance.

8. Exercise leaders serving as role models and activity leaders are vital for short term attendance and overall

effectiveness of training programs for obese clients. Peer support also improves the degree of adherence.*

9. Efforts should be made to identify individuals with the need for more exercise leadership and structured activity than others. Questioning will help identify those people who are more dependent. Frequently these subjects will stop exercising when supervised sessions end.

10. Try to provide a gymnasium facility whenever possible. This includes use of a locker room, exercise clothing, shower facilities, and other conveniences. If this is not possible, some kind of home-base setting should be identified. By providing this atmosphere, a routine is established and emphasized.

11. Complete records of clients adherence and compliance to prescribed exercise should be maintained. Daily workout logs should include feedback on subjective perceptions, training heart rate during exercise, complaints, injuries, and general comments. Entries may be recorded by exercise leaders or the subject as a personal diary.

12. Teach the clients how to accurately monitor their resting and exercise pulse rates. The concept of achieving the prescribed training heart rate must be fully explained so the subject learns how to monitor and pace his intensity during exercise so that cardiovascular improvements may be safely realized.

13. Monitor exercise heart rate more frequently at the beginning of a program. In addition, note perceived exertion, as the client learns to identify his individual responses. Over time, monitoring can become less frequent [23].

14. Interval training and modifications should be considered as alternatives to continuous exercise. In cases where subjects experience difficulty in maintaining the duration component of their exercise prescription, intermittent phases of

*See B. A. Franklin, Exercise program compliance: improvement strategies. In *Behavioral Management of Obesity*, edited by J. Storlie and H. A. Jordan. (New York: Spectrum Publications, 1984).

intense and low activity can be introduced. This is particularly important when increasing from a low level to a more intense activity. For example, progression from a walking to a jogging routine or rehabilitation from an injury are situations where interval training is appropriate.

15. Advocate self-help activities, such as calisthenics, to be performed at home on a regular basis as a supplement to aerobic activities. In addition, increased daily activities should be emphasized along with regular exercise, e.g., walking to do errands, taking stairs, parking a distance from a destination, and limiting the use of labor saving devices. All of these minor changes promote a positive step toward an active lifestyle.

16. Educate clients that physical work capacity and exercise tolerance often improve at a faster rate than actual weight loss [29]. These improvements may be recognized with improved performance over standard distances, increased stamina with consistent intensity, and overall feeling of improved fitness as the heart rate remains in its training zone.

17. Establish training goals and program progressions to meet those goals for each client [38]. Record entries so that recognition of personal achievement can be acknowledged by exercise leaders and peers.

18. Supervised training sessions should be conducted in peer group settings for best cost effectiveness. This allows efficient use of exercise leaders and provides peer support.

19. Clients should be accurately weighed on the same scale at regular intervals. These weights should be recorded on a graph and used to monitor progress. It is important that a staff member be on site during weigh-in sessions to provide encouragement and advice.

20. Many clients will be following calorically restricted diets along with their exercise prescription. Diets of mixed composition are recommended. Both moderate [39] and extremely obese [29] subjects can perform endurance exercise of moderate intensity while maintaining a diet low in carbohydrates. Monitor the tolerance of individuals with periodic questioning or reporting in regard to diet and overall energy level.

REFERENCES

1. Braunstein, J. J. Management of the obese patient. *Medical Clinics of North America*, *55*, 391–401, 1971.
2. Bray, G. A. Clinical management of the obese adult. *Postgraduate Medicine*, *51*, 125-129, 1972.
3. Harris, M. B., and Halbaur, E. S. Self-directed weight control through eating and exercise. *Behavior Research and Therapy*, *11*, 523-529, 1973.
4. Schteingart, D. E., Foss, M. L., Lampman, R. M., Short, M., Buntman, H., Michael, R., and McGowan, J. Obesity—a multidisciplinary approach to management. In Howard, A. *Recent Advances in Obesity Research*, Newman Publishing, London, pp. 304-307, 1975.
5. Stuart, R. B. Exercise prescription in weight management: advantages, techniques and obstacles. *Obesity/Bariatric Medicine*, *4*, 16-24, 1975.
6. Hursh, L. M. Exercise in weight reduction. *Nebraska Medical Journal*, *61*, 158-160, 1976.
7. Wertz, S. H., and Wertz, R. L. Exercise and diet as therapeutic aids in weight reduction and subsequent control. *American Corrective Therapy Journal*, *21*, 122-130, 1976.
8. Thompson, J. K., Jarvie, G. L., Lathey, B. B. and Cureton, K. J. Exercise and obesity: etiology, physiology, and intervention. *Psychological Bulletin*, *91*, 55-79, 1982.
9. Wing, R. R. and Jeffery, R. R. Outpatient treatments of obesity: a comparison of methodology and clinical results. *International Journal of Obesity*, *3*, 261-279, 1979.
10. Oscai, L. B. The role of exercise in weight control. In Wilmore, J. H., *Exercise and Sports Science Reviews*, Academic Press, New York, pp. 103-123, 1973.
11. Woo, R., Garrow, J. S., and Pi-Sunyer, F. X. Effects of exercise on spontaneous calorie intake in obesity. *American Journal of Clinical Nutrition*, *36*, 470-477, 1982.
12. Epstein, L. H. and Wing, R. R. Aerobic exercise and weight. *Addictive Behaviors*, *5*, 371-388, 1980.
13. Buskirk, E. R., Thompson, R. H., Lutwak, L., and Whedon, G. D. Energy balance of obese patients during weight reduction: influence of diet restriction and exercise. *Annals of New York Academy of Science*, *110*, 918-940, 1963.
14. Buskirk, E. R. Obesity: a brief overview with emphasis on exercise. *Federation Proceedings*, *33*, 1948-1951, 1974.
15. Metropolitan Life Insurance Company. Frequency of overweight and underweight. *Statistical Bulletin*, *41*, 4-7, 1960.

16. American College of Sports Medicine. *Guidelines for Graded Exercise Testing and Exercise Prescription.* Lea and Febiger, Philadelphia, pp. 2-5, 1980.
17. American Heart Association Committee on Exercise. *Exercise Testing and Training of Apparently Healthy Individuals: A Handbook for Physicians.* American Heart Association, New York, 1972.
18. American Heart Association Committee on Exercise. *Exercise Testing and Training of Individuals with Heart Disease or at a High Risk for its Development: A Handbook for Physicians.* American Heart Association, Dallas, 1975.
19. Cooper, Kenneth H. *The Aerobics Program for Total Well-Being.* M. Evans and Company, Inc., New York, 1983.
20. Mathews, D. K. and Fox, E. L. *The Physiological Basis of Physical Education and Athletics.* W. B. Saunders Company, Philadelphia, 1976, pp. 503-511.
21. Naughton, J. Cardiac rehabilitation: principles, techniques, applications. In Amsterdam, E. A., Wilmore, J. H., and DeMaria, A. N. *Exercise in Cardiovascular Health and Disease.* Yorke Medical Books, New York, pp. 364-376, 1977.
22. Pollock, M. L., Wilmore, J. H., and Fox, S. M. The exercise prescription. *Health and Fitness through Physical Activity.* John Wiley and Sons, New York, pp. 117-177, 1978.
23. Foss, M. L. Exercise prescription and training program for obese subjects. In Bjorntorp, P., Cairello, M., and Howard, A. N. *Recent Advances in Obesity Research: III.* John Libbey & Co., London, 1981.
24. Bjorntorp, P. Exercise in the treatment of obesity. *Clinics in Endocrinology and Metabolism, 5,* 431-453, 1976.
25. Franklin, B., Buskirk, E., Hodgson, J., Gahagan, H., Kollias, J., and Mendez, J. Effects of physical conditioning on cardiorespiratory function, body composition and serum lipids in relatively normal weight and obese middle-aged women. *International Journal of Obesity, 3,* 97-109, 1979.
26. Gwinup, G. Effects of exercise alone on weight of obese women. *Archives of Internal Medicine, 135,* 676-680, 1975.
27. Lewis, S., Haskell, W. L., Wood, P. D., Manoogian, N., Bailey, J. E., and Periera, M. B. Effects of physical activity on weight reduction in obese middle-aged women. *American Journal of Clinical Nutrition, 29,* 151-156, 1976.
28. Leon, A. S., Conrad, J., Hunninghake, D. B., and Serfass, R. Effects of a vigorous walking program on body composition and carbohydrate and lipid metabolism of obese young men. *American Journal of Clinical Nutrition, 32,* 1776-1787, 1979.

29. Foss, M. L., Lampman, R. M., and Schteingart, D. E. Extremely obese patients: improvements in exercise tolerance with physical training and weight loss. *Archives of Physical Medicine and Rehabilitation*, *61*, 119–124, 1980.
30. Goodman, C. and Kenrick, M. Physical fitness in relation to obesity. *Obesity/Bariatric Medicine*, *4*, 12–15, 1975.
31. Moody, D. L., Kollias, J., and Buskirk, E. R. The effect of a moderate exercise program on body weight and skinfold thickness in overweight college women. *Medicine and Science in Sports*, *1*, 75–80, 1969.
32. Pollock, M. L., Miller, H. S., Janeway, R., Linnerud, A. C., Robertson, B., and Valentino, R. Effects of walking on body composition and cardiovascular function of middle-aged men. *Journal of Applied Physiology*, *30*, 126–130, 1971.
33. Girandola, R. N. Body composition changes in women: effects of high and low exercise intensity. *Archives of Physical Medicine and Rehabilitation*, *57*, 297–299, 1976.
34. Moody, D. L., Wilmore, J. H., Girandola, R. N., and Royce, J. P. The effects of a jogging program on the body composition of normal and obese high school girls. *Medicine and Science in Sports*, *4*, 210–213, 1972.
35. Foss, M. L., Lampman, R. M., Watt, E., and Schteingart, D. E. Initial work tolerance of extremely obese patients. *Archives of Physical Medicine and Rehabilitation*, *56*, 63–67, 1975.
36. Karvonen, M. J., Kentala, E., and Mustala, O. The effects of training on heart rate. A longitudinal study. *Annales Medicinae Experimentalis et Bilogiae Fenniae*, *35*, 305–315, 1957.
37. American College of Sports Medicine. Position statement on the recommended quantity and quality of exercise for developing and maintaining fitness in healthy adults. *Medicine and Science in Sports*, *10*, vii–x, 1978.
38. Foss, M. L., Lampman, R. M., and Schteingart, D. E. Physical training program for rehabilitating extremely obese patients. *Archives of Physical Medicine and Rehabilitation*, *57*, 425–429, 1976.
39. Phinney, S. D., Horton, E. S., Sims, E. A., Hanson, J. S., Danforth, E., Jr., and LaGrange, B. M. Capacity for moderate exercise in obese subjects after adaptation to hypocaloric ketogenic diet. *Journal of Clinical Investigation*, *66*, 1152–1161, 1980.

6

Exercise Concerns and Precautions for the Obese

Merle L. Foss

INTRODUCTION

The primary foci of this chapter are the special needs of obese clients who are being considered for exercise testing and training and the associated concerns and precautions. Awareness on the part of exercise leaders and clinicians (referred to herein as exercise therapists) is an important step to the development and vending of safe, yet effective exercise training programs that are prudent and within current established standards of practice in the U.S. A concerted effort has been made to present this material, such that problems are both identified and practical solutions suggested. To this end, the most common problems encountered while working with obese persons in exercise settings are mentioned with the hope that exercise therapists will be more conscious and can circumvent some potentially troublesome areas which could lead to injury and possibly malpractice or liability litigation.

While an effort has been made to relate as much content to the scientific literature as possible, the reader should be aware that some practical suggestions are based on empirical observations made during the experience of working with moderately obese students and extremely obese patients in a university setting. The reader also should be aware that both subject groups were eating calorically restricted mixed diets during the periods of their exercise testing and training. Moderately obese college-age students were following self-monitored intakes of approximately 1000-1500 kcal/day (daily deficits of about 700 kcal) whereas extremely obese patients were on semi-starvation diets of 400-600 kcal/day with vitamin and mineral supplements. The data from these studies do not therefore reflect an "exercise alone" approach to the treatment of obesity, but rather the use of exercise as an important, if not essential, adjunct therapy in the rehabilitation process. This presentation format coincides with the author's bias that while the impact of exercise "alone" on fat reduction is of significant academic interest, exercise produces the best results when used along with calorically restricted diets and behavior modification therapies [1]. Therefore, the rehabilitation process operates best as a combined positive treatment force which concomitantly impacts the patient.

Figure 1 addresses the question of what constitutes optimum therapy for resolution of obesity when it is viewed as a widespread health problem. While we currently lack a definitive answer to this question, there is evidence supporting basic therapies that focus on dietary intake, physical activity, and modification of associated behaviors. These therapies hold the best promise for the greatest number of obese citizens in our multicultural society. Other aspects of optimal therapy might include a variety of self-help activities, psychological support form therapists or peers, and a periodic evaluation of progress (i.e., checking in with an authority figure or support

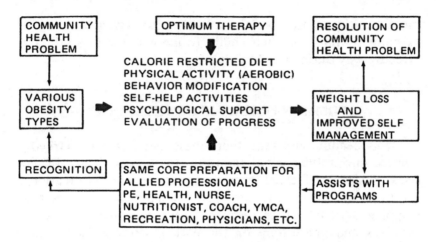

Figure 1. Optimum therapy for resolving obesity as a community health problem.

person so that body weight loss or gain is documented). The model suggests that optimal therapeutic regimens can better be defined for various types of obese persons (consider age, gender, pre-adolescent, maturity-onset, hyperplastic, hyper-trophic obesities) if allied professionals from a variety of specialty fields have been exposed to the same core preparation in the general areas of dietetics/nutrition, exercise physiology, and behavioral psychology. As indicated, these professionals may come from a wide variety of backgrounds including physical educators, health educators, nurses, nutritionists, coaches, YMCA and health spa employees, recreation therapists, and physicians from many sub-specialties, to name a few. While the goal that all professionals working in any common area have the same basic core preparation and exposures is idealistic and most likely unattainable, the aspects of optimum therapy that hold implications for exercise can be identified and integrated. An attempt will therefore be made to interrelate the matters of physical activity, exercise behavior modification, self-help exercises, psychological support training, and evaluation of training progress with exercise concerns and precautions as stated earlier. This approach will hopefully leave the reader

more sensitive to the special needs of obese participants as well
as more confident in their ability to use exercise in a safe and
effective way during weight reduction.

COMMON PROBLEMS OF THE OBESE

It is readily apparent that obese persons are markedly
stressed during their initial exposures to exercise. They display
outward signs of flushed faces, perspiration, labored breathing,
shortness of breath, and are easily fatigued to the point of
stopping activity. These responses have signalled a need for
concerns and precautions on the part of exercise leaders and
may have been the primary reason for earlier recommendations
that obese persons should not participate in vigorous physical
activity [2]. It is now better understood that the obese can
safely participate in beneficial exercise programs provided that
some of their common problems are considered and steps taken
to circumvent, or correct them [3].

Table 1 lists several of the most common problems of obese
clients which may limit their exercise performance. Each of
these are discussed in some detail followed by practical
solutions for dealing with each problem. In some cases the
"solution" is in the form of a registered concern since there
may be little that actually can be done about the problem,
while in other cases specific precautionary and correctional
procedures are suggested.

**Table 1. Common Problems of Obese Clients
Which May Limit Their Exercise Performance**

Heat intolerance	Orthopedic pain
Hyperpnea-dyspnea	Local muscular weakness
Movement restriction	Balance-anxiety

HEAT TOLERANCE

During exercise obese persons are less tolerant to ambient heat and to internal body heat buildup than their leaner counterparts [4]. This is manifested in the early onset of facial vasodilation seen as flushed skin, in early profuse sweating, in complaints about being "too hot," and expressions of generalized fatigue. Since much of this problem relates to the insulative and overload effects of excess fat layers, there is little that can be done as an immediate direct solution. Many patients apparently undergo some rapid temperature regulation adaptations or lessened perceptions of exertion as they continue training since they are clearly more tolerant of their exercise induced heatloads.

Their heat intolerance also improves with weight loss, so getting them safely through the first few sessions is the most difficult challenge to the exercise therapist. During these early sessions, participants should be encouraged to wear proper clothing that minimizes heat stress. Although many patients do not want to expose their bodies, they should wear conventional gym clothing such as shorts, light weight cotton tee shirts, and low cut sweat sox. Tight fitting, closely knit nylon or rubberized fabrics should not be permitted, and long sleeved shirts or long legged trousers and slacks discouraged.

Other procedures that help to counteract the heat intolerance of exercising obese patients include concern for the environment, the type and intensity of the workout, and the availability of drinking water. Exercise rooms must be maintained at cool temperature settings. Avoiding the hottest part of the day is important when conducting outdoor exercise sessions. If participants are riding stationary bicycles, fans should be available to provide cooling air currents. Swimming in cool water provides a fine form of activity during hot and humid days. There is evidence that the obese also tolerate the performance of other exercises better in cool water [5].

When exercising in the heat, participants will achieve their training heart rate prescriptions at a lower intensity than when performing the same activity on a cool day. This indicates that adjustments in terms of pace or lap speed can be made to lower the workout intensity. It is also sensible to allow more frequent rest periods on hot days, and to encourage drinking plenty of cool water before, during, and after exercise sessions.

As a final precautionary measure, alert patients to the early signs and symptoms of heat stress so they can monitor themselves and others. The exercise therapist should instruct participants to immediately report *any* sensations such as headaches, throbbing or light headedness, dizziness, nausea, or unsteadiness. A more ideal procedure is to have them sit on the floor and summon the attention of the exercise leader should any of these symptoms arise.

BREATHING

A problem common to exercising obese persons is dyspnea, or difficulty in breathing, and hyperpnea or very fast breathing [6–8]. Both are experienced more often during initial exercise sessions and tend to subside, as described for heat intolerance. These sensations can be very distressful to participants, leading to fear and anxiety about their well-being. The associated perceptions of exertion may be so strong that the participant will express a desire to stop activity saying "I can't go any longer or further, etc." These complaints should be acknowledged and the participant encouraged to stop for a short rest period. During this time the therapist should monitor the rate and type of breathing pattern, recording the time required to recover a comfortable level of breathing. The recovery period can be used to educate the participant about the strong perceived exertion messages that relate to rapid breathing. It is important to emphasize that they will eventually gain control and become more tolerant of these symptoms. Therapists should also determine whether the participant is breathing through both open mouth and nose during exercise. Breathing through the nose only limits oxygen uptake and causes problems for some people.

Some positions assumed during traditional calisthenic and stretching exercises contribute to the breathing difficulties of many obese participants. For example, toe touching from standing, chair-seated, or floor-seated positions with static holding compresses the chest cavity and inhibits breathing. This position is a common flexibility exercise for the back and legs, but initially it should be avoided or minimized. The same precaution is indicated for any exercises which involve trunk flexion for prolonged periods such as inverted bicycling, or rolling back from a supine lying position and placing the legs overhead. Conversely, dynamic exercises which require static efforts for brief periods of time, (e.g., bent-knee sit ups, alternate toe touching from a standing position, or forward bending from a seated position) are considered desirable from two standpoints. First, conventional exercises provide necessary flexibility and strength training. Secondly, this type of exercise briefly exposes the participant to relatively uncomfortable positions, so tolerance can be improved.

MOVEMENT RESTRICTION

Extremely obese patients frequently have restrictions in movement due to excessive layering of fat. This usually means that exercise therapists need to modify many traditional calisthenic exercises so they can be performed adequately and safely. The movement restriction is apparent in both joint range of motion and the speed with which limbs can be moved. It is usually quite easy to develop a modified form of any exercise which is within the performer's capabilities and allows them to progress as they lose weight. An example of this is the modified pushup which at first can be performed from a standing, forward-leaning position against a wall, then a standing, leaning position against a sturdy desk top, then from a crawling position against the floor, from a straight-back, knee-touching position against the floor, and finally from a straight-body, toes-touching position against the floor. It is very important to emphasize these modifications in group exercise settings.

ORTHOPEDIC PAIN

Obese clients frequently complain about orthopedic-related pain in their spine, hips, knees, and ankles [9]. Further, a higher incidence of arthritis exists in obese populations [10]. It is questionable whether or not the incidence and its impact on the ability of obese clients to safely pursue and complete exercise sessions is significantly different than non-obese participants. Most of the common problems are quite prevalent in both groups. In any case, a thorough initial evaluation of orthopedic status is warranted to document previous and current incidents of inflammation, swelling, pain, injury, restricted range of motion, etc.

Back Pain

Most chronic upper and lower back problems are initially apparent and subside with improved fitness and weight loss. A reasonable strategy for lessening spinal discomfort is to intersperse low back stretching exercises with the aerobic workouts as a rest period (Figure 2). These exercises are considered to be effective for alleviating acute episodes of low back pain. The supine position also provides support for the upper back region when the shoulders and upper spine are forced to a more

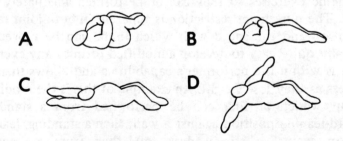

Figure 2. Static stretching exercise to alleviate lower (A and B) and upper (C and D) back pain.

flattened position. The client is in a safe, nonstressful posture which is well-tolerated compared to standing, bench-seated or floor-seated positions as mentioned earlier. The exercises can be performed with the head flexed forward toward the chest or in a backward extended position. The client should hold knees to the chest for as long as comfortable for a maximum of 15 seconds and repeat each hold position three times (position A, Figure 2). Between each repetition they should return to the position of slightly bent knees with heels resting on the floor (position B, Figure 2). During this part of the exercise, the hands should be pressed downward on the abdomen, while the pelvis is thrust upward for a 15 second static hold. This maneuver involves simultaneously contracting abdominal muscles to flatten the stomach, relaxed stretching of the lower back muscles, and forceful contraction of the buttocks muscles to complete the pelvic thrust.

If the source of pain is primarily in the upper back, the client should be instructed to lie flat on their back with knees partially bent, feet flat on the floor and arms extended along the floor at shoulder level (position C, Figure 2). After flattening the upper spine, neck, and shoulder blades against the floor, the client should hold this position for a count of 15 seconds. In this same position, with elbows on the floor, arms should be raised overhead and held for 15 seconds. This sequence can be repeated 3 times (i.e., 3 sets).

After performing these stretching exercises, the client should continue with the scheduled workout. The advantages of doing corrective exercises at the time of complaint are that individuals begin to associate their chronic problem with skeletomuscular causes and are provided with a ready solution that helps in most cases. Further, self-help activities, which can be practiced on a daily basis for prophylactic benefits, are introduced. Through this approach, the exercise program can be continued and eventually tolerance to chronic back problems will increase, until the pain gradually subsides and disappears.

Ankles, Knees and Hips

A somewhat different approach should be used for complaints of pain in the ankles, knees or hips as these problems tend to be more acute [11] rather than chronic. Further, the symptom may relate more to exercise strain resulting from intense workouts, inappropriate facilities and equipment, or a poor selection of footwear. This is not to say that some complaints do not relate to old injuries, chronic inflammation, or degenerative arthritic processes, but a distinction should be made. Mainly, if a client complains of localized pain during an exercise session or before beginning a subsequent workout, the problem frequently can be related to overstrain caused by biomechanical factors.

Before initiating an exercise program, advise clients to purchase high quality, well-fitted shoes that are designed for the type of activity chosen. Examples are: jogging shoes for walking, jogging, or running; court shoes for recreational games such as volleyball or racquetball; and bicycling shoes for stationary or road biking. While it is difficult to argue that a client couldn't safely pedal a bike for prolonged periods while wearing court or jogging shoes, a close inspection of each type of shoe reinforces this recommendation. Biking shoes are light in weight, flexible, and provide a minimum of lateral ankle support, but have a very stiff, thin sole that protects the bottom of the foot from prolonged localized pedal compression forces. On the other hand, jogging shoes have thicker soles constructed of materials which cushion against heavy repetitive strike forces, which occur during each contact of the foot with the surface and sturdy sidewalls which provide needed lateral support to the ankle.

Participants should not be allowed to wear shoes of poor quality in any exercise session because of the risk of injury. Supply clients with adequate information to be properly fitted, by a reputable footwear vendor, with high quality and comparatively inexpensive shoes that will protect them from injury. It is usually helpful to provide the client with the names of popular manufacturers and models to aid in the selection process. Further, the salesperson should be informed that they will be engaging in relatively lower intensity activities, like walking or jogging, for prolonged periods; thus, a heavier, thicker soled, more durable shoe is desirable. If exercise leaders are working with large numbers of clients, it may be efficacious to prepare a list of appropriate models that should work well based on recent publications and simply check off some recommendations dependent on the type of activity to be performed. In any case, don't allow clients to begin exercise programs with poor footwear because the risk of injury to ankles, knees, or hips is too great, resulting in potentially unnecessary set backs in the rehabilitation process. Often, an early injury is the only negative message that the client needs to prompt the conclusion, "I guess I really am too heavy to exercise" and "I don't think I'll do it any more." Actually, the shoes were at fault.

It is not uncommon for an exercising obese client to develop a localized injury to their lower limbs, despite proper footwear. Sometimes these injuries can be related to facilities and equipment such as jogging on a concrete surface, walking around a small banked track, or riding a poorly maintained stationary bicycle. When a client complains of injuries to specific regions, the cause may be identified from records or questions pertaining to the activities being performed or those performed on prior days. For example, repeated jogging sessions on a hard surface like concrete sidewalks may explain pain in the front of one or both shins called "shin splints." Likewise, fast walking around a short, sharply banked track may place undue strain on the ankle of the "inside" leg. Pain in the knee-cap region of one or both legs may be due to a stationary bicycle which provides a pulsative resistance requiring a powerful pumping action during leg extension rather than a smoothly turning flywheel. The watchword is, when acute injuries occur, look for a logical explanation. This operational guideline is particularly helpful for episodes of localized joint pain which show up unexpectedly. This is in contrast to acute trauma, related to slipping, twisting, or falling actions. If its a new complaint and the client denies any knowledge of cause, look to overstrain related to equipment or facilities as a probable explanation.

General Guidelines for Treating Orthopedic Problems

Attempts to alleviate pain problems related to overstrain are often made using a trial and error method. After deciding on the most probable cause, it is best to adjust only one variable at a time unless it is clear that several factors are contributing. After the initial adjustment is made, it is important to allow adequate time for improvement.

During the foregoing trial and error procedure it is important to remember that the client has incurred some trauma to localized tissues and that this trauma is the cause of the pain. Subsequent exercise sessions at the same combination of intensity and duration will aggravate the condition, even if the most appropriate correctional adjustment has been made. For this reason, it is appropriate to reduce the intensity and duration of exercise required of the client. Note that exercise has not been stopped altogether and should not be unless the pain becomes worse. A strategy of attempting to have the client "work through" the problem is advocated, but at the same time correctional adjustments have to be made and the total amount of exercise must be reduced to encourage a healing process. The educational benefits of this experience for the clients are usually significant and help to intelligently manage future problems of pain and trauma which may occur.

Athletic Injuries

The final matter to consider in the area of orthopedic pain is joint problems that are clearly related to abrupt trauma caused by actions, such as slipping, twisting, falling, hyperextension of joint, or impact forces. These can all be categorized as "athletic injuries" that occur during exercise and should be treated as such [9]. That is, the same conservative treatment approaches that are used to rapidly return competitive athletes to activity should be used with clients who incur injuries during rehabilitative or preventative exercise sessions. These standardized procedures include:

1. initial examination of the injured body area;
2. questioning the injured person and documenting the cause of the injury;
3. immobilizing, applying compression bandages and elevating the injured region;
4. applying cold as needed to control any swelling;
5. deciding whether x-ray evaluations for possible bone fractures are needed (these are usually taken if heavy impact forces were received, if popping or cracking noises are heard at the moment of injury, or if pain is excessive and persistent, and are often taken if there is any doubt at all about the possibility of fractures);
6. embarking on a rather immediate program of injury rehabilitation which could include a variety of therapies depending upon the setting and connections with athletics training rooms, physical therapy departments, or private clinical services.

If the injury is severe, the client should be treated by qualified professionals who work with athletic related trauma. Professionals in this area will suggest appropriate therapies and monitor the client's progress throughout the rehabilitation process. If the injury is not severe, the client may be directed toward a program of self-rehabilitation. This program would include the application of ice to the injured region two to three times daily for maximum periods of 20 minutes during the first few days after injury. After several days, when the injury has stabilized, inflammation is gone, and swelling is reduced, the same routine may be used with hot water soaks. Another therapy is to alternate cold and hot treatments for 15 minutes each. After these cold or hot treatments, the injured area should be massaged and manipulated through the joint's range-of-motion by actively contracting muscles and by applying forces (hands, arms, leaning postures) in various directions around the injured joint. The noninjured joint can be used as a comparative gauge for the amount of impairment in joint range-of-motion. In this process, the joint is forced to the point of pain or resistance, allowed to relax and adjust to the position, and then forced to move a bit further. This latter position should be held for 15 seconds followed by free joint movement and massage and the procedure repeated 3–5 times.

Although it is sometimes possible and even recommended that clients perform exercise as part of their injury rehabilitation, extremely good sense must govern such decisions. This represents a departure from the strategy described earlier where clients would be encouraged to perform the same type of activity at reduced intensity and duration in order to sort out problems related to equipment, facilities, and biomechanical factors. In the case of severe injuries, the client might perform strengthening exercises to protect the other tissues during a long rehabilitation process, while avoiding the type of activity that caused the injury. It may be desirable to prescribe swimming, weight training, stationary biking, or other programs of activity during recovery.

On the other hand, if the injury is not severe, and the client can tolerate minimal sensations of pain, continuing the original exercise program in combination with self-rehabilitation therapies will be beneficial. Good sense is the key to selecting the best approach, but a major consideration is that injured clients can frequently continue to exercise by simply changing modalities. When the time comes for severely injured clients to reinitiate a physical activity program, they should begin slowly and progressively. For example, if an individual is ready to return to jogging after a rehabilitative phase on a stationary bicycle for 40 minute sessions, it would be best to initially walk for a 5 minute period, leading up to 15 minutes of continuous walking as a substitute for part of the bicycle workout. Once 40 minutes of walking can be managed, 5 to 15 minutes of jogging should replace part of the walking, until it is possible to comfortably jog for 40 minutes. This process should take about 12 weeks (Table 2) but allows a safe return to the preferred activity.

Once again, the client should have learned some valuable lessons from the injury rehabilitation experience:

1. it is possible and desirable to exercise even when injured,
2. other types of exercise can be substituted in the event of injury when it is no longer possible to perform a favorite activity, and
3. the rehabilitation process, which may involve both professional and self-care, is more clearly understood.

MUSCLE WEAKNESS

Localized weakness due to poorly developed and atrophied muscles is quite common in obese clients, especially in the upper body. Females are particularly subject to this problem.

Table 2. Example of Progressions for Returning to Jogging After Severe Ankle Injury

- 40 minutes jogging
- severe injury to ankle
- no leg activity for 3 sessions (1 week)
- 10 min biking for 3 sessions (1 week)
- 20 min biking for 3 sessions (1 week)
- 30 min biking for 3 sessions (1 week)
- 40 min biking for 3 sessions (1 week)
- 15 min biking, 5 min walking × 2 for 3 sessions (1 week)
- 10 min biking, 10 min walking × 2 for 3 sessions (1 week)
- 5 min biking, 15 min walking × 2 for 3 sessions (1 week)
- 40 min walking for 3 sessions (1 week)
- 15 min walking, 5 min jogging × 2 for 3 sessions (1 week)
- 10 min walking, 10 min jogging × 2 for 3 sessions (1 week)
- 5 min walking, 15 min jogging × 2 for 3 sessions (1 week)
- 40 minutes jogging

Total weeks = 12
Lost workouts = 0
Modalities used = 3

Conversely, the lower body and leg regions have undergone a slow, progressive strength adaptation in order to bear an increased body weight. Exercise leaders should attend to devising strength development programs for obese clients according to individual needs. While it would be advisable to conduct strength tests of localized muscle groups, it is possible to devise strength training programs without administering these tests. In most cases, a lack of upper body strength (particularly in the arms, shoulder girdle, and abdomen) will limit performance in weight-supported calisthenics, like modified push-ups.

Weaknesses can be corrected with modified calisthenics as part of a group exercise session and as self-help activities to be performed at home. Calisthenic exercise can be included as a special component of the group activity class or they can be interspersed into the aerobic portion of the workout as recovery intervals. For example, after each 5 laps around the gym, the participants engage in a number of modified sit-ups, modified push-ups, leg lifts, etc. In either case, the reason for performing each exercise should be explained in relation to specific muscles used. Time should also be spent teaching the proper form for conducting the exercises, possible sequences of progression, and any precautions that should be followed.

Additional and faster improvements in upper body strength can usually be made if clients also begin progressive resistance exercise (weight training) programs using either machine or free weights. Such programs should be viewed as supplemental and not as a substitute for the calisthenics–aerobics activities previously described. The self-help calisthenics and aerobic exercises are the mainstays in that they can be performed without special equipment. In cases where weight training programs are requested or warranted to improve motivation, it is critical that clients be instructed on the following:

1. proper lifting technique,
2. lifts that will benefit them most,
3. basic principles of strength and endurance training,
4. proper breathing techniques to avoid the valsalva maneuver,

5. general safety,
6. a need to use spotters for overhead lifts of free weights (military press, bench press).

Many obese clients are eager to try weight training and require little convincing that it will benefit them. Some of the benefits include:

1. predictable improvement in body self-image;
2. muscular development which can counteract loose, saggy skin after body fat loss;
3. protection of lean body mass during fat weight loss;
4. improvement of chronic low back pain condition due to stronger abdominal and back muscles;
5. improved basic survival potential because arms and shoulders are stronger;
6. common reports that weight training participants enjoy the feelings of "getting stronger" and the associated improvements in their self-esteem.

BALANCE

Another problem of obese clients which might limit their exercise performance is anxiety related to their sense of balance. This problem is much more common in extremely obese clients [12] than in the moderately obese, but it is wise to demonstrate concern in either case. For example, some extremely obese clients express a fear of falling and not being able to get up, particularly in an open room without furnishings to use as supports. Lesser obese clients express more concern about moving rapidly and performing quick movements in a variety of activities because they have never "done them before."

Most obese clients have reasonably good motor coordination for basic movements such as walking, jogging, and running, so anxiety about balance appears unrelated to poor coordination. Anxiety seems more related to excessive body mass and concern over the effects of momentum (mass times velocity) which contributes to losing balance during unfamiliar movements. Special exercises to improve balance and dispel fears can be included in training sessions; however, most problems will naturally subside after a few sessions. Initially, question clients about previous balance problems and determine if they have fear of falling. In cases of extreme anxiety it is advisable to provide longer orientation periods, comprised of low intensity exercise and specially adapted activities which utilize handrails, padded floor areas, or other safe support structures. These sessions should include instruction on techniques for getting up from an open floor area without assistance if that is a problem.

DISEASES, METABOLIC DISORDERS
AND COMPLICATIONS OF THE OBESE

Obese clients who have known diseases or metabolic disorders present special problems when becoming involved in a safe, effective exercise program [13-15]. Some of the more common conditions are listed in Table 3.

Cardiovascular Disease

The classification of cardiovascular disease includes any disease state which compromises the pumping action of the heart or effective circulation of blood to any region of the

Table 3. Diseases and Complications of Obese Requiring Precautionary Concern or Exercise Program Modification

• Cardiovascular disease	• Pulmonary hypertension
• Arterial hypertension	• Ionic disbalance
• Diabetes	• Orthostatic hypotension
Ulcerations	
Hypoglycemia	
Ketoacidosis	

body. This encompasses a variety of disorders, most of which are related to atherosclerosis. Typical symptoms are chest pain (angina), leg pain (intermittant claudication), and reduced work tolerance.

While controversy still persists over whether obesity, in and of itself, should be viewed as a risk factor for cardiovascular disease and premature heart attacks, it has been positively correlated to diabetes mellitus through epidemiological studies. Obese persons have more hypertension and diabetes. Further, in developing these conditions, the obese are at higher risk for incurring significant cardiovascular disease at an earlier age. The obese client with one or more cardiovascular risk factors (e.g., arterial hypertension, hypercholesterolemia, or cigarette smoking) with or without the presence of secondary risk factors, should be considered at higher risk for developing coronary heart diseases. Obese clients presenting with one or more risk factors should, therefore, be given a graded exercise stress test with ECG monitoring for purposes of medical screening and development of an exercise prescription. (See Chapter 5 "Exercise Testing and Training for the Obese.") Certainly those with known heart disease should have a graded exercise stress test if at all possible so that subsequent intensity assignments can be made below the level at which any signs and symptoms of ischemic heart function, intermittant claudication, or abnormal blood pressure responses occur.

Ideally, it is best if obese clients with cardiovascular complications exercise in supervised/monitored settings; however, this might not be possible considering the magnitude of the epidemic problem. Alternatively, they must be instructed about the following:

1. proper quantity and type;
2. safeguards related to the activity;
3. how to monitor their pulse rate and adjust exercise intensity to achieve, but not exceed, their THR;
4. how to record selected information about their exercise response and progress, perceptions of strain and exertion, any aches and pains.

Table 4. Generalized Low Intensity (60%) Target Heart Rate
Assignments Dependent on Clients' Age

Age	MHR[a]	RHR[b]	CR[c]	THR[d]
20	200	75	125	150
30	190	75	115	144
40	180	75	105	138
50	170	75	95	132
60	160	75	85	126
70	150	75	75	120

[a]Estimated maximum heart rate by 220 – age.
[b]Resting heart rate estimation.
[c]Cardiac reserve by MHR-RHR.
[d]Target heart rate by 60% of CR + RHR.

By reviewing these records, the exercise therapist can become familiar with the exercise response of each client and better plan reasonable and safe progressions. In general, three strategies are important when exercising obese clients who have cardiovascular complications or hypertension. These recommendations are: (1) the intensity of activity should be decreased; (2) longer orientation periods are necessary to introduce safety precautions; (3) close monitoring by trained staff is critical throughout the exercise program.

It is important to emphasize that the client's personal physician should be included as part of the weight reduction team. The physician can provide initial screening for heart disease and identification of metabolic disorders that relate to obesity before referral to qualified exercise specialists for the development of appropriate activity programs. It is important for the physician to retain responsibility for primary care of the obese cardiac patient during weight reduction. This team approach requires frequent communication within the management team. It is particularly important when weight loss programs last several months to a year or more. Further, adjustments in one or more therapies frequently impact effectiveness of other therapies. Interdisciplinary teamwork is, therefore, critical.

Diabetes Mellitus

Obese clients present special needs and challenges to the exercise therapist. Three major concerns are:

1. ulcerations
2. hypogylcemia, and
3. ketoacidosis (Table 3)

There are a number of lesser concerns that are not as life threatening. These have been documented elsewhere and the interested reader is encouraged to peruse these descriptions [16–18].

Diabetics have compromised peripheral circulation, which is manifest in a loss of sensation in the extremities, especially their feet. For example, a fold in a stocking may not be perceived and result in a significant blister in a diabetic client. Healing is slow because of this poor circulation, so the risk of an ulceration developing into a gangrene infection is possible. Surgical excision or even amputation could be the end result. With such serious consequences, it is essential that diabetic–obese clients be educated about proper footwear, footcare, and inspection of the soles of their feet for "hotspots" after each exercise session. Furthermore, the exercise therapist should instruct the client to monitor any area of their body where abrasions might occur during exercise. For example, the insides of their thighs often become chaffed by rubbing together during bicycling, walking, or jogging. Hands or feet may become sore from riding a stationary or road bicycle. Frequent inspection and careful cleansing of these areas, followed by the application of powders or lotions, is the first line of defense against serious complications.

The insulin-dependent diabetic patient will need to more closely monitor their blood glucose levels during exercise, since they risk the possibility of becoming hypoglycemic or developing severe ketoacidosis. Both of these conditions reflect an inadequate management of exogenous insulin in relation to food intake and energy expenditure during recreational or occupational activities.

In the case of hypoglycemia, blood sugar levels drop because food intake is too low or insulin levels are too high. This situation is complicated by exercise which promotes the clearance of glucose from the blood stream as it circulates to actively contracting muscles. If the most recent insulin dose has been injected into the region of active muscle, its clearance from the depot site is rapid, resulting in a sharp drop in blood glucose levels. This condition is referred to as marked or severe hypoglycemia, hypoglycemic shock, or insulin shock. In contrast, blood sugar levels are elevated (hyperglycemia) during ketoacidosis because there is inadequate insulin for glucose uptake. The cells switch to lipid metabolism in order to meet basal energy requirements. Ketone bodies are produced during cellular metabolism of free fatty acids as a source of fuel. The blood pH drops due to the acidity of the ketone bodies, hence the name ketoacidosis. When ketoacidotic diabetics begin to exercise, free fatty acid metabolism is stimulated to meet the energy demands of activity, so ketoacidosis is exacerbated by exercise. In the ketoacidotic state the problem is inadequate insulin, while hypoglycemia results from too much insulin. It is clear that exercising a diabetic requires a careful balance of exogenous insulin with food intake.

Since nerve cells cannot function well in a glucose-deprived or highly acidic environment, both of these complications lead to disorientation, faulty judgement, ataxia, and possible coma. The outcome could be tragic if either ketoacidosis or hypoglycemia occurred while the client was exercising alone in sparsely traveled areas. Some safeguards for protecting insulin-dependent diabetics against the problems of severe hypoglycemia or ketoacidosis during exercise are obviously required. Since obese insulin-dependent diabetics are likely to be following calorically restricted diets, the application of these safeguards is complicated.

The schedule of exercise should be coordinated with the insulin administration to avoid blood insulin peaks. This peak will depend on whether short- or long-acting insulin is being used so the type of insulin needs to be considered. The insulin should be injected into the abdominal region away from muscle masses used in activity. Small snacks prior to exercise can be planned into the overall caloric intake. Sugar sources in the form of sugar cubes, hard candy, or fruit juices must be available to meet emergency hypoglycemic situations. In fact, exercising diabetics should establish the habit of carrying hard candy when involved in activity. Subjective responses to assigned exercise should be closely monitored to find a proper balance between the insulin dosage, caloric requirements, and tolerance for exercise.

Ideally, blood insulin and glucose and urine glucose and ketone levels should be assayed during the initial phases of an exercise program. After an optimal combination is determined and exercise training is underway, it is important to periodically reassess insulin requirements. Frequently, insulin needs diminish by 25–40%, or in some cases, are eliminated in response to physical conditioning.

To avoid problems of severe ketoacidosis, the obese insulin-dependent diabetic should not exercise on days when the morning urine sample indicates glucosuria and ketonuria. This precaution will prevent complications until insulin and blood glucose have stabilized in response to a new exercise program. Regulation of insulin dosage must be under the control of the primary care physician. This is another health team concept, using the patient/client as an important and integral controller of individual health care. In addition to these precautionary measures, standard guidelines for programs apply to obese-diabetic clients.

Other Disease Factors

Pulmonary hypertension, ionic disbalance, and orthostatic hypotension will be discussed in a cluster because all of these metabolic conditions have been frequently described in the scientific literature as complications of obesity, which may contraindicate exercise therapy. While precaution is warranted, the actual risk is not as significant as the literature might indicate. For example, reports exist of exercise-induced pulmonary hypertension in obese patients, but this does not manifest itself in outward signs of compromised exercise tolerance at low to moderate intensities [19]. A similar impression is noted for complaints of muscle cramps which may be related to ionic disbalance. Since these problems were encountered by extremely obese patients who were following severely restricted caloric intakes without mineral supplements, the incidence would be less among moderately obese clients who are consuming adequate calories to prevent electrolyte imbalances. The problem is best alleviated by clients adjusting their intake of salt.

Orthostatic hypotension during floor exercise settings, however, has only been observed in formerly obese patients immediately after they have finished a bout of strenuous exercise [20]. In these few cases, the problem was managed by reducing the intensity of the exercise sessions until the client regained orthostatic stability. A safeguard against these latter conditions is to keep complete records of symptoms and complaints experienced during or between exercise sessions. These notations can prevent more serious future complications. Improved screening and exercise training techniques will minimize the risk of these problems.

SUMMARY

Figure 3 summarizes the most notable responses to exercise that occur in the obese and the areas of greatest concern. Keeping these factors in mind should allow therapists to work more competently and confidently with obese clients who are slightly, moderately, or extremely obese. Some guidelines for categorizing the severity of obesity and the predisposition to coronary heart disease lead to intelligent management of the inherent risks of exercising the obese.

Obese persons can safely participate in exercise programs when certain precautions are taken. This is not to say that involvement is without risk or that problems and injuries will not occur. The frequency of problems and the overall

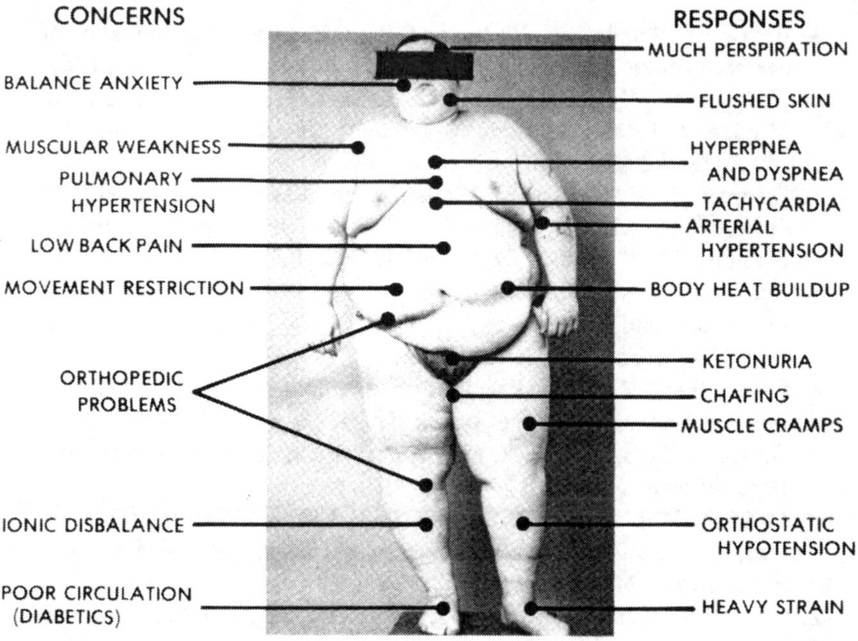

Figure 3. Summary of notable exercise responses and concerns of the obese.

inherent risks can be minimized. Thus, exercise will serve as an important adjunct therapy in the war against pandemic obesity.

REFERENCES

1. Schteingart, D. E., Foss, M. L., Lampman, R. M., Short, M., Buntman, H., Michael, R., and McGowan, J. Obesity—a multidisciplinary approach to management. In *Recent Advances in Obesity Research*, ed. A. Howard, pp. 304-307. London: Newman, 1975.
2. Cooper, K. H. Guidelines in the management of the exercising patient. *J.A.M.A. 211*:1663-1667, 1970.
3. Foss, M. L. Exercise prescription and training programs for obese subjects. In Bjorntorp, P., Cairella, M., and Howard, A. N. (eds.) *Recent Advances in Obesity Research: III*. John Libbey and Co., London, 1981.

4. Bar-Or, O., Lundegren, H. M., and Buskirk, E. R. Heat tolerance of exercising obese and lean women. *J. Appl. Physiol.* 26:403–409, 1969.
5. Sheldahl, L. M., Buskirk, E. R., Loomis, J. L., Hodgson, J. L., and Mendez, J. Effects of exercise in cool water on body weight loss. *Int. J. Ob.* 6:29–42, 1982.
6. Dempsey, J. A., Redden, W., Balke, B., and Rankin, J. Work capacity determinants and physiological cost of weight supported work in obesity. *J. Appl. Physiol.* 21:1815–1820, 1966.
7. Bray, G. A., Whipp, B. J., Koyal, S. N., and Wasserman, K. Some respiratory and metabolic effects of exercise in moderately obese men. *Metabolism* 26:403–412, 1977.
8. Farebrother, M. J. B. Respiratory function and cardiorespiratory response to exercise in obesity. *Br. J. Dis. Chest.* 73:211–229, 1979.
9. Goodman, C., and Kenrick, M. Physical fitness in relation to obesity. *Obesity/Bariatric Med.* 412–415, 1975.
10. Levinson, M. L. Obesity and health. *Prep. Med.* 6:172–180, 1977.
11. Gwinup, G. Effect of exercise alone on weight of obese women. *Archs. Intern. Med.* 135:676–680, 1975.
12. Foss, M. L., Lampman, R. M., Schteingart, D. E., and Watt, E. Initial work tolerance of extremely obese patients. *Archs. Phys. Med. Rehabil.* 56:63–65, 1975.
13. Buskirk, E. R. Obesity: a brief overview with emphasis on exercise. *Fed. Proc.* 33:1948–1951, 1974.
14. Dempsey, J. Exercise and obesity. In *Sports Medicine*, ed. A. J. Ryan and F. I. Allman, Jr., pp. 557–593. New York: Academic Press, 1974.
15. Björntorp, P. Exercise in the treatment of obesity. *Clinics in Endocrinology and Metabolism* 5:431–453, 1976.
16. Berg, K. The insulin-dependent diabetic runner. *The Physician and Sportsmedicine* 7:71–79, 1979.
17. Diabetes and exercise—a roundtable discussion. *The Physician and Sportsmedicine* 7:47–61, 1979.
18. Koivisto, V. A. and Sherwin, R. S. Exercise in diabetics—therapeutic implications. *Postgraduate Med.* 66:87–96, 1979.
19. Alexander, J. K. Obesity and cardiac performance. *Am. J. Cardiol.* 14:860–865, 1964.
20. Foss, M. L., Lampman, R. M., and Schteingart, D. E. Extremely obese patients: improvements in exercise tolerance with physical training and weight loss. *Archs. Phys. Med. Rehabil.* 61:119–124, 1980.

Index

Lightning Source UK Ltd.
Milton Keynes UK
UKOW05f0848031014

239556UK00002B/97/P